The
Dimensions
of Health
CONCEPTUAL MODELS

John R. Hjelm, PhD
North Park University
Chicago, Illinois

JONES AND BARTLETT PUBLISHERS
Sudbury, Massachusetts
BOSTON   TORONTO   LONDON   SINGAPORE

World Headquarters

Jones and Bartlett Publishers
40 Tall Pine Drive
Sudbury, MA 01776
978-443-5000
info@jbpub.com
www.jbpub.com

Jones and Bartlett Publishers
Canada
6339 Ormindale Way
Mississauga, Ontario L5V 1J2
Canada

Jones and Bartlett Publishers
International
Barb House, Barb Mews
London W6 7PA
United Kingdom

Jones and Bartlett's books and products are available through most bookstores and online booksellers. To contact Jones and Bartlett Publishers directly, call 800-832-0034, fax 978-443-8000, or visit our website, www.jbpub.com.

Substantial discounts on bulk quantities of Jones and Bartlett's publications are available to corporations, professional associations, and other qualified organizations. For details and specific discount information, contact the special sales department at Jones and Bartlett via the above contact information or send an email to specialsales@jbpub.com.

Production Credits
Acquisitions Editor: Shoshanna Goldberg
Senior Associate Editor: Amy L. Bloom
Editorial Assistant: Kyle Hoover
Production Manager: Julie Champagne Bolduc
Production Assistant: Jessica Steele Newfell
Associate Marketing Manager: Jody Sullivan
V.P., Manufacturing and Inventory Control: Therese Connell
Composition: Glyph International
Cover Design: Kristin E. Parker
Photo Research Manager and Photographer: Kimberly Potvin
Assistant Photo Researcher: Bridget Kane
Cover Image: © amygdala imagery/ShutterStock, Inc.
Printing and Binding: Malloy, Inc.
Cover Printing: Malloy, Inc.

Library of Congress Cataloging-in-Publication Data
Hjelm, John R.
  The dimensions of health : conceptual models / John R. Hjelm.
     p. ; cm.
  Includes bibliographical references and index.
  ISBN 978-0-7637-5609-3 (alk. paper)
  1. Health behavior. 2. Health. I. Title.
Thygerson, Steven M. II. Thygerson, Justin S. III. Title.
  [DNLM: 1. Attitude to Health. 2. Health Behavior. 3. Health. W 85 H478d 2010]
  RA776.9.H54 2010
  613--dc22
                                                                    2009033026
6048

Printed in the United States of America
13 12 11 10 09   10 9 8 7 6 5 4 3 2 1

Contents

Preface

I had an epiphany while attending graduate school in the late 1980s. I was introduced to the idea that health is multidimensional. Our culture has a tendency to equate thinness and overall physical appearance with health rather than considering a person's overall lifestyle and behavior. This book attempts to illustrate that health incorporates the whole person, and examines the complicated and holistic nature of health.

As I began teaching undergraduate health classes, I noticed that many textbooks presented a multidimensional view of health, but did not develop a foundational, holistic approach. Since then I have studied the writings of others and tried to assimilate their ideas into my own concept of health. For several years my classes also worked to develop their own models for each dimension. Eventually, it became clear that a more concentrated attempt to integrate the dimensions was needed. *The Dimensions of Health: Conceptual Models* is an outgrowth of my research and teaching. It incorporates the multidimensional concept of health and is intended to be a tool to help students understand the five dimensions of health: physical, social, emotional, intellectual, and spiritual. The models proposed are intended to stimulate discussion among professionals and students. They should prompt critical thinking, but should not be viewed as the final answer to the question, "What is health?"

Chapters 2 through 6 of this book review definitions, descriptions, and models of one of the five dimensions of health. The concluding chapter emphasizes the overlapping, interacting nature of each of the dimensions. The overall aim of this book is to provide insights for both introductory and higher-level health courses, to stimulate professionals to engage in serious discussions about what is meant by *health*, and to motivate others to develop more models for each of the dimensions. Such work can help us move forward on a path toward healthful living.

CHAPTER 1 ▶

The Concept of Health

Health is the thing that makes you feel that now is the best time of year.

—Franklin P. Adams

It is of value to think of health as that condition of the individual which makes possible the highest enjoyment of life, the greatest constructive work and that shows itself in the best service to the world.

—Jesse Feiring Williams, 1930

Introduction

People are unsure about what it means to be healthy. Most would agree that a man with cancer is not healthy. They may not be so sure about someone with no friends or no purpose in life. A variety of students responded to several statements about the meaning of health. A sampling of their thoughts is presented in **Box 1.1**.

This sample of responses demonstrates diverse ideas about health. Many students focus on bodily function. Others focus on lifestyle issues such as safer sex and avoiding drugs. Exercise and diet are also common emphases. Some students define health by what it is not. They believe health is not being obese or not being sick. Some take a more psychological perspective. They focus on happiness or mental function. A few look into the future, suggesting that health is related to living longer. Many topics are typically included in the study of health (see **Box 1.2**). This book, however, is not a study of the facts of health. Instead, it seeks to help you answer the bigger question, "What is health?"

Box 1.1 Statements About Health

Health is satisfying your body's needs in order to prolong life.

Healthy people are self-aware and self-motivated.

Healthy people live longer and enjoy life more.

Health is personal balance.

Health means taking care of your body.

Healthy people have more energy.

Health is physical fitness.

Health means living life to the fullest.

Health is physical, mental, and emotional wellness.

Healthy people make positive lifestyle choices.

Healthy people don't get sick.

Health means treating your body with respect.

People are healthy when they exercise and eat well.

Healthy people look good.

Health means your physical, spiritual, and mental wellness.

Health is being free from disease.

Healthy people like sports.

Healthy people exercise, stay drug free, and use safer sex.

Box 1.2 Topic Areas in Health

Birth control

Cancer

Cardiovascular disease

Environment

Health care

Nutrition

Physical Fitness

Relationships

Sexuality

Sexually transmitted disease

Stress management

Substance abuse

Violence and victimization

Weight management

Health is a concept. Concepts are ideas or thoughts that bring together different elements resulting in a cohesive whole. The list of responses from students indicates there are many thoughts about health. This book provides a framework you can use to more fully develop your personal concept of health.

Psychiatrist M. Scott Peck (1987) helps explain why there are so many opinions about the meaning of health. He believes that humans can "define or adequately explain only those things that are smaller than we are" (p. 59) and that there are many "things" too big for us to understand fully. According to Peck, these "things" include God, goodness, evil, and love. Health is another one of those "things." It is so large and multifaceted that there is no adequate one-sentence definition. We can, however, examine the *idea* of health by studying descriptions, illustrations, and models that give us different perspectives on the whole concept. This is also true of each of the components of health, which we will call *dimensions*. Our goal is to begin to understand these complicated ideas and see how the information fits together.

Our understanding of health is still evolving. The concept of health has changed significantly over the last 150 years. Early ideas equated health with the absence of disease and later with hygiene (Donatelle, 2006, p. 6). "Unsickness" indicated good health. With the discovery of pathogens, people realized they could adopt certain behaviors to prevent disease. This ushered in the era of hygiene—people washed regularly and avoided drinking dirty water. The focus was still on caring for the body, however; the concept of health was limited to the physical dimension.

In the 1940s the World Health Organization (WHO) proposed the idea of health as a multidimensional concept. This new definition stated that "health is a state of complete physical, mental, and social well-being and not merely the absence of disease or infirmity" (WHO, 1948). This landmark definition is still widely used. Its publication was a turning point in the evolution of what it means to be healthy. "Health" was no longer limited to the physical dimension. The WHO definition recognized that humans are more than just their bodies.

By the late 1950s Halbert Dunn, a physician, was emphasizing the idea that health was a positive or optimal state of being, not just a neutral condition. He coined the term *wellness* to represent this positive state of health. His radio talks were published in a book titled *High Level Wellness* (Dunn, 1961), and his notion of health as vitality and zest for life began to receive more attention. Dunn's perception of health as "high level" functioning is apparent in his description of wellness. "There are . . . times when you are fairly alive with the glow of good health—with wellness. Alive clear to the tips of your fingers. You have energy to burn. You tingle with vitality. At times like these, the world is a glorious place!" (Dunn, p. 2).

Most health educators today agree that health is multidimensional. An informal review of college textbooks shows that five dimensions are present in virtually all models (Breuss & Richardson, 1994; Byer & Shainberg, 1995; Donatelle, 2006; Edlin & Golanty, 2007; Floyd, Mimms, & Yelding, 2008; Hales, 2009; Insel & Roth, 2004; Payne & Hahn, 2002). Those dimensions are the physical, social, emotional, intellectual, and spiritual. Some of these authors suggest additional dimensions. Hales, Insel and Roth, and Donatelle all incorporate environmental health in their models. Occupational health is also included by some (Breuss & Richardson; Byer & Shainberg; Edlin & Golanty). This book contends that environmental health is a part of social and spiritual health and that occupational health may incorporate aspects of social, intellectual, and emotional health. These dimensions are not sufficiently distinctive; therefore, they are not included as separate dimensions. **Figure 1.1** illustrates the model of health used in this book.

Some writers take a very different approach. Travis and Ryan (1988) propose a Wellness Energy System. Their model is based on the idea of energy flow, where energy flows into the body via three avenues (eating, sensing, and breathing) and exits via nine paths (self-responsibility, moving, feeling, sex, transcending, finding meaning, communication, playing and working, thinking). However, a closer examination of these paths reveals a relationship with the more traditional dimensions of health. For example, thinking is related to the intellectual dimension and transcending is related to the spiritual dimension.

Balog (2005), a health educator at SUNY Brockport, provides a view contrary to the prevailing wisdom. He believes that the entire movement toward health as

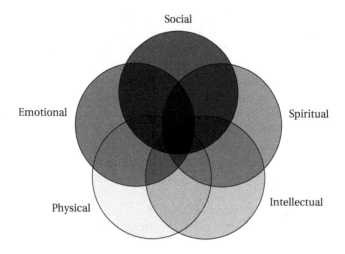

Figure 1.1 The Dimensions of Health

multidimensional is wrong. Balog insists that emotional, social, and spiritual factors can contribute to health, but that they are not health. They are related to the "good life." He also contends that health resides within the individual. According to this thinking, such things as relationships cannot be health, because they occur outside the body. Balog contends that health is purely physical and is "defined by how well the body is functioning in accordance with its natural design" (p. 270).

Although opinions differ regarding the components of health, it is clear that most agree with the idea that health includes several dimensions. This division of health into components helps us study and discuss the topic. However, it is important to remember that the dimensions interact and overlap (see Figure 1.1). They complement each other to form the whole person. In fact, the word *health* comes from an Old English word meaning "wholeness" (Barnhart, 1988; Breuss & Richardson, 1994). As you study the following chapters, watch for overlaps between dimensions. You may find as you read about one dimension that some ideas about it seem relevant in another dimension as well. That is the nature of health.

Similarly, changes in one dimension affect the other dimensions. For example, a person who begins an exercise program to lose weight (physical) may also improve his or her self-esteem (emotional). A college student studying philosophy to fulfill university requirements (intellectual) may discover meaning in life, a purpose for living (spiritual). When you have the flu (physical), you probably don't feel like spending time with your friends (social).

Byer and Shainberg (1995) believe that health is a "cultural concept"; that is, different cultures have different beliefs about just what health is. This is an important consideration. As you read this book, consider your own culture, upbringing, and religious beliefs. Evaluate the information in the book in the context of your

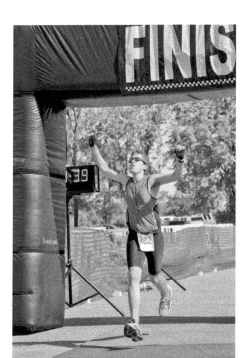

The dimensions of health are overlapping and interacting. This runner may be experiencing the emotion of elation even though his body is exhausted.

history and values. Use them to fine tune your personal definition and model of health. Several perspectives are presented here to stimulate your thinking.

A Word about Conceptual Models

A model of health was presented earlier in this chapter. It includes five overlapping, interacting dimensions. Models for each of the five dimensions of health will be presented in later chapters. But what are models and how are they useful?

Perhaps you built models when you were a child. Many children enjoy assembling model cars or animals. These figures are not real, but they are similar to the real thing. A model car has an engine and doors and a steering wheel. Models of birds are often life size and carefully painted to match the colors of real birds. The models provide information about real cars and real birds. Children can learn about reality from them.

In the same way, conceptual models are developed to represent reality. They provide mental maps that attempt to provide information logically and realistically (American Institutes for Research, 2004). They may represent objects or ideas.

Studying models
helps understand
reality.

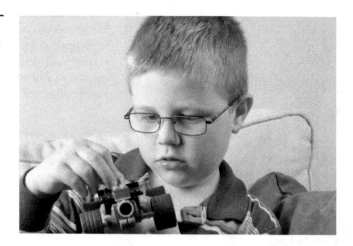

The best models are simple, accurate, and easy to understand. They organize information and represent the real thing (Jarvelin & Wilson, 2003). A model "provides a working strategy, a scheme containing general, major concepts and their interrelations" (Jarvelin & Wilson). This is the goal of this book. It organizes knowledge and ideas about each of the five dimensions of health and identifies relationships between them.

A multidimensional model of health forms the foundation of this book. It assumes that the five dimensions adequately include and integrate the necessary aspects of the whole person. This component model showing the five dimensions will help you develop your own understanding of health. As you study the models for each dimension, reflect on the intersections that exist.

Organization of the Chapters

The next five chapters examine each of the five dimensions of health. The chapters follow the same format. The "Introduction" traces the etymology of the word and provides context for the study of that dimension. "Definitions and Descriptions" provides examples of how experts think about that dimension. The "Models" section presents two or more models developed by scholars and professionals in health education and related disciplines. The next section proposes "Characteristics" of people who exhibit health in that dimension and attempts to answer the questions, "How do I recognize this dimension of health?" and "What can I do to improve my health in this dimension?" "A New Model of . . ." concludes each chapter with the author's attempt to assimilate the information and presents a model built on the thinking and writing of previous writers.

What is health? Although this book does not pretend to provide the final answer to that question, it does provide a variety of answers and perspectives that may be useful to you as you try to answer this very important question.

Ignore your health . . . and it will go away!

Discussion Questions

1. Write your personal definition or description of health. How does it compare and contrast with your classmates' definitions?
2. How can you recognize a healthy person?
3. Why is it difficult to agree on a single definition of health?
4. How are models useful for understanding complicated ideas? Give examples of models you have used.

References

American Institutes for Research. (2004). *WAI web site usability test.* Retrieved February 4, 2006, from http://www.air.org/concord/wai/conceptual.html

Balog, J. E. (2005). The meaning of health. *American Journal of School Health, 36*(5), 266–271.

Barnhart, R. K. (Ed.). (1988). *The Barnhart dictionary of etymology.* New York: H.W. Wilson.

Breuss, C. E., & Richardson, G. E. (1994). *Healthy decisions.* Madison, WI: Brown & Benchmark.

Byer, C. O., & Shainberg, L. W. (1995). *Living well: Health in your hands* (2nd ed.). New York: HarperCollins College.

Donatelle, R. J. (2006). *Access to health* (9th ed.). San Francisco: Pearson Benjamin Cummings.

Dunn, H. (1961). *High level wellness.* Arlington, VA: R.W. Beatty.

Edlin, G., & Golanty, E. (2007). *Health and wellness* (9th ed.). Sudbury, MA: Jones and Bartlett.

Floyd, P. A., Mimms, S. E, & Yelding, C. (2008). *Personal health: Perspectives and lifestyles* (4th ed.). Belmont, CA: Thomson Wadsworth.

Hales, D. (2009). *An invitation to health.* Belmont, CA: Wadsworth Cengage Learning.

Insel, P. M., & Roth, W. T. (2004). *Core concepts in health* (9th ed.). Boston: McGraw-Hill.

Jarvelin, K., & Wilson, T. D. (2003). On conceptual models for information seeking and retrieval research. *Information Research, 9*(1). Retrieved February 24, 2006, from http://informationr.net/ir/9-1/paper163.html

Payne, W. A., & Hahn, D. B. (2002). *Understanding your health* (7th ed.). Boston: McGraw-Hill.

Peck, M. S. (1987). *The different drum: Community making and peace.* New York: Simon & Schuster.

Travis, J. W., & Ryan, R. S. (1988). *The wellness workbook* (2nd ed.). Berkeley, CA: Ten Speed Press.

World Health Organization. (1948). Official records of the World Health Organization, no. 2. Proceedings and final acts of the international health conference held in New York from 19 June to 22 July 1946. New York: United Nations WHO Interim Commission.

CHAPTER 2 ▶

Physical Health

> *The body will have health only if each cell regards the needs of the whole body.*
>
> —Paul Brand, *Fearfully and Wonderfully Made*, p. 60

> *The body cannot be ignored. The body is me, I am my body.*
>
> —George Sheehan, 1992

Introduction

Jacob lost 25 pounds and thinks he is healthy. Kim has been lifting weights and looks toned. She thinks she is healthy. Historically, health has been associated with the condition of the body. Physical health in its simplest form refers to efficient functioning of the body or "the biological integrity of the individual" (Greenberg, 1985, p. 403). The word *physical* is from the Latin word *physica*, which originally meant "things relating to nature" (Chantrell, 2002). Early usage in English was related to "medicinal." The first recorded use associating the word *physical* directly with the body was in 1780 (Barnhart, 1988). Present usage refers to the material universe or the human body. Physical focuses on matter. Corporeal and somatic are synonyms. We could just as easily use the phrase *corporeal health* or *somatic health*.

Health often is still used in a way that emphasizes the body. People say things like, "You look healthy. Have you lost weight?" We assume that being thin indicates health, whereas being fat is a sign of poor health. One of the components of health-related fitness is body composition. Sometimes we even equate the appearance of a suntan with health. In fact, just the opposite is true. A tan indicates

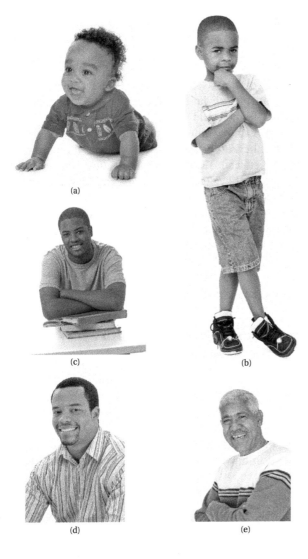

People change
physically throughout
their lives.

(a)

(c)

(b)

(d)

(e)

that the skin has been damaged. When we recover from a cold or the flu, we say, "It feels good to be healthy again!" These examples all equate bodily function or appearance with health.

The body changes throughout a lifetime. Human development is a discipline that studies these changes; however, you don't have to be an expert to recognize that the body of a newborn is quite different from that of a child. The brain also grows and develops, allowing higher levels of thinking; Swiss psychologist Piaget has identified a developmental sequence for cognitive abilities (Ormrod, 1995). During puberty the body develops further so that reproduction is possible. The elderly are generally recognizable by further changes in their bodies that result in a regression of physical capabilities. Reproduction and hard physical labor may no longer be possible.

The body is an important aspect of who we are. Some people believe that humans were created in the "image of God" (Genesis 1:26). This image is reflected in the whole person (Sherwin, 1991). Physician Paul Tournier reminds us that it is through our bodies that we are "in the world" (Sarano, 1966).

Some scientists view the body as a machine. They propose that physiology is best understood in this context because it allows us to compare the human body to other machines (Foss & Keteyian, 1998). For example, fluid movement due to pressure can be compared to the cooling system of a car. Movement of body parts can be described using principles of levers. Although this approach certainly has value, it is limiting. The body adapts and even becomes more efficient with use, whereas machines wear out. The body is an important part of who we are. Physician Jacques Sarano (1966) sums this up: "The body is more than a commodious instrument that I could do without: my body is myself, the man who I am" (p. 49). The physical is one of the five dimensions of health. The body's function plays an essential role in each person's total well-being.

Definitions and Descriptions of Physical Health

Dianne Hales (2009), a respected author of health textbooks, envisions a physical health continuum with premature death at one end and wellness in which you "feel and perform at your very best" (p. 5) at the other end. She suggests that we need to take steps away from illness to become healthier. Physical health seems to be avoidance of something negative.

Donatelle (2005) includes characteristics such as "body size and shape, sensory acuity and responsiveness, susceptibility to disease and disorders, body functioning and physical fitness, and recuperative abilities" (p. 4) in her concept of physical health. She also suggests that the ability to perform activities of daily living is a part of physical health.

Process rather than characteristics is the focus of descriptions by both Insel and Roth (2004) of Stanford University and Edlin and Golanty (2007). They suggest that reaching a high level of physical health requires such activities as healthful eating, regular exercise, avoiding harmful habits, making responsible decisions about sexual activity, learning about disease, preventing injury, and getting regular medical examinations.

Breuss and Richardson (1994) are well-known health educators and writers. They focus on efficient functioning, resistance to disease, and the "physical capacity to respond appropriately to varied events" (p. 5).

Physical fitness is emphasized in some descriptions of physical health. Floyd, Mimms, and Yelding (2008) list the components of health-related physical fitness in their description of physical health. They believe that physical health encompasses cardiovascular endurance, flexibility, muscle strength and endurance, and body composition.

Psychiatrist M. Scott Peck (1987) offers an uncomplicated view of physical health. He writes that it "involves caring effectively for our physical body" (p. 289). He focuses on physical fitness, proper diet, and getting enough rest.

Dr. Michael Roizen (1999) believes that we should think of physical health as the "prevention of aging" rather than the more common approach of disease prevention. He suggests that when we take care of our bodies, time slows down; that is, we have more time to do what we want and need to do.

Payne and Hahn (2002), health educators from Ball State University, emphasize the importance of anatomy and physiology in personal development. They cite physical characteristics such as body weight, visual ability, strength, coordination, endurance, susceptibility to disease, and recuperative power as key physical attributes.

Alters and Schiff (2009) focus on physiology of body systems. They suggest that physical health "relates to the overall condition of the organ systems." They believe that we can recognize poor health by symptoms such as fever, rashes, fatigue, and headaches. When the systems are functioning efficiently the "individual feels well and is free of disease" (p. 3).

These descriptions by experts provide differing perspectives on physical health. Some of the descriptions emphasize function; others focus on a long life or physical fitness. The common denominator, of course, is the body.

Models of Physical Health

Formal models of physical health have not been developed; however, we can use the perspectives of several disciplines to examine physical health. Efficient functioning of the body is one characteristic of physical health. Balog (2005) limits his definition of overall health to the physical dimension and writes that it is "defined by how well the body is functioning in accordance with its natural design" (p. 270). So we must consider what the body is designed to do and how it can function efficiently. The following perspectives could be considered models of physical health.

Physical Fitness Model

Physical fitness is typically viewed from two perspectives. Motor or skill-related fitness includes components that are particularly valuable for performance. Athletes might be concerned with agility, reaction time, balance, coordination, power, and speed. Health-related fitness incorporates cardiorespiratory endurance, muscle strength, muscle endurance, flexibility, and body composition (American College of Sports Medicine [ACSM], 2006).

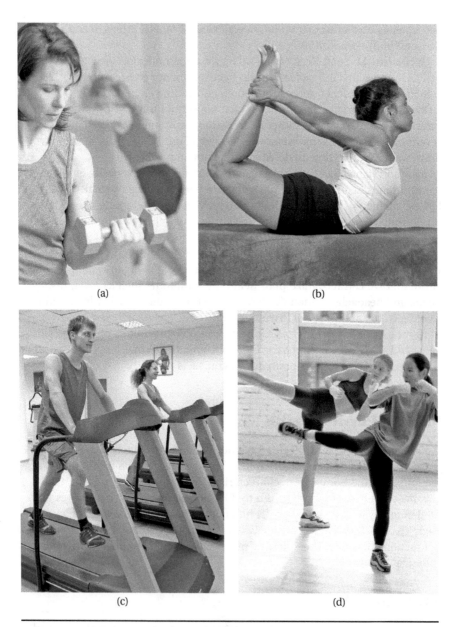

Components of physical fitness: (a) strength, (b) flexibility, (c) cardiorespiratory fitness, and (d) balance.

The components of health-related fitness enhance the body's functioning in ways conducive to health. Fit people reduce their risk of disease (primarily through cardiorespiratory fitness) and improve their ability to perform activities of daily living (through strength, endurance, and flexibility). Balance also contributes to activities of daily living.

Motor Development Model

Motor development is one component of human development. It focuses on your ability to move and manipulate objects. Basic skills such as walking, running, striking, and throwing develop early in life. Specialized skills such as hurdling, driving a golf ball, and playing the piano occur later and require specific training and practice. Thus high levels of physical health would be characterized by highly organized, complex motor skills (Payne & Isaacs, 2005). Development of basic skills is natural for most children. Development of specialized sports skills depends on opportunity, practice, and motivation.

Motor development includes both growth and maturation. Growth is simply an increase in size. Height and weight increase during childhood. This is growth.

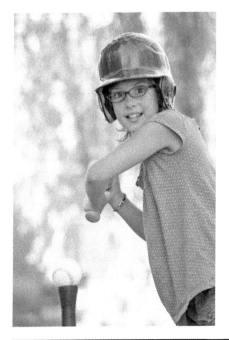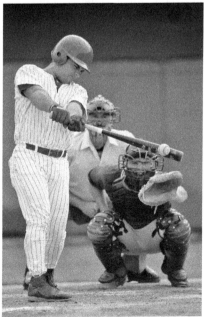

Motor skills such as striking develop over time.

Maturation refers to functional changes. Puberty is an obvious example of maturation. The reproductive system matures rapidly during adolescence and the individual becomes capable of producing offspring.

Gabbard (2004) describes the developmental continuum. Infants learn rudimentary behaviors such as grasping, crawling, and walking. These are early voluntary movements. Children then learn fundamental movements such as running, jumping, twisting, kicking, and throwing. During later childhood they learn sport skills; that is, fundamental movements become specialized as children develop interests in specific sports. Kicking skills are refined by soccer players, for example. During the growth spurt of adolescence, skills are refined and the individual's larger size and muscle mass provide new opportunities for motor skills. Adults reach peak performance levels in their late twenties, and this is followed by a period of regression throughout adulthood and into late adulthood.

Body Systems Model

Biologists and physicians might view physical health from the perspective of physiology. The body is composed of systems that contribute particular functions to the work of the body (Fox, 1999). A list of these systems appears in **Table 2.1**.

A detailed description of this model of health is beyond the scope of this text. Therefore, we will examine one system as an example. The leading cause of death in the United States is cardiovascular disease; thus, the circulatory system would be an appropriate example to study. The circulatory or cardiovascular system is composed of the heart and blood vessels. As mentioned in Table 2.1, its primary function is transport of blood and lymph. Blood is pumped throughout the body carrying nutrients and byproducts of metabolism. The blood should move efficiently and have healthy levels of cholesterol, hemoglobin, red blood

Table 2.1 Systems of the Human Body

Body System	System Function
Integumentary	Protection and thermoregulation
Nervous	Regulation of other body systems
Endocrine	Secretion of regulatory hormones
Skeletal	Movement and support
Muscular	Movements of the skeleton
Circulatory	Movement of blood and lymph
Immune	Defense of the body against pathogens
Respiratory	Gas exchange
Urinary	Regulation of blood volume and composition
Digestive	Breakdown of food
Reproductive	Continuation of the human species

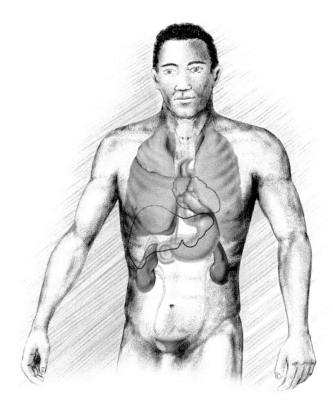

The body system model evaluates physical health by studying systems such as the cardiovascular and respiratory systems.

cells, and white blood cells (to name a few components). The heart needs to contract regularly and forcefully to move the blood. Health (or efficiency) of the cardiovascular system can be determined in a variety of ways:

▶ Resting heart rate can be monitored by individuals. Generally, a lower heart rate is healthier. This would indicate that enough blood is being pumped per beat.

▶ Resting blood pressure is typically measured at the doctor's office, although home monitors can also be purchased. Guidelines for healthy systolic and diastolic pressure have been published (ACSM, 2006).

▶ Graded exercise tests assess the cardiovascular system's response to acute exercise. Heart rate and blood pressure are monitored. An electrocardiogram provides information about the electrical activity of the heart. The electrical activity indicates whether the myocardium is contracting appropriately.

▶ Blood tests are often used to ensure that the blood itself is healthy. These tests assess levels of cholesterol, triglycerides, and other blood components.

▶ Echocardiograms use ultrasound to provide a real-time view of heart structures, including the valves.

Box 2.1 Cardiovascular Fitness
Average resting heart rate is 72 beats per minute.
Average resting blood pressure is 120/80 mm Hg.
Normal total cholesterol level is less than 200 mg/dL.

Box 2.1 provides typical recommendations for variables of cardiovascular fitness.

Tests are available to assess the health of other body systems as well.

If physical health is characterized by efficient functioning of the body, a question must be asked: functioning for what? Several possible answers come to mind: functioning for pleasure, for service, for worship, for procreation, and so on. Any model of physical health must address this question. Of course, there may be several appropriate answers because the body is used for different purposes at different times.

Characteristics of Physically Healthy People

Dr. Breslow, Dean Emeritus at UCLA and a public health pioneer, developed the "Seven Healthy Habits" (Sheehan, 1992). These habits were proposed years ago, but are still useful today:

1. Eat a good breakfast.
2. Don't eat between meals.
3. Maintain your weight.
4. Don't smoke.
5. Drink moderately.
6. Get a good night's sleep.
7. Exercise regularly.

Dr. Breslow focused on process rather than product. He asked what we should do to reach the goal of physical health.

Dr. Michael Roizen (1999), an internist and author of *Real Age*, suggests that we should think of physical health as the prevention of aging. We need to take care of our bodies. There are three crucial aspects that contribute to physical health. First, we must care for our arteries. Roizen writes, "You are as young as your arteries" (p. 7). Second, we must protect the immune system. And finally, we must control social and environmental factors such as stress and secondhand smoke.

Using the fitness model described earlier, we could describe the physically healthy individual as one who is physically fit. This person would score well on tests of cardiorespiratory endurance, muscle strength, muscle endurance, flexibility, and body composition. He or she would have adequate levels of fitness to complete activities of daily living and have energy left to enjoy recreational activities.

A New Model of Physical Health

The information presented above does not lead to an obvious model of physical health. A model must consider both efficiency and natural design (Balog, 2005). Runner and physician George Sheehan (1992) writes that we express ourselves through our bodies. We do this in three ways, and those three modes—movement, thought, and procreation—form the basis of our model of physical health. The systems of the body serve these three activities.

Movement

Movement is a crucial characteristic of the human body. Humans are born to move. It is natural from the moment of birth, and even in the womb. The muscular and skeletal systems work together to produce movement; however, other systems also contribute. The digestive system provides energy for motion, the cardiovascular system transports nutrients to the muscles, and the respiratory system provides the oxygen necessary for metabolism. Movement allows us to work, create, play, serve, and reproduce.

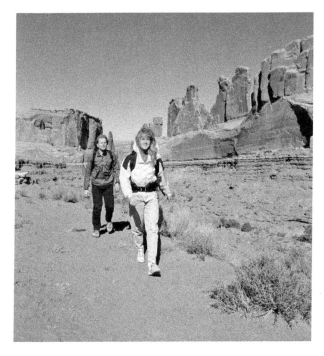

Efficient movement is one component of physical health. Humans use movement to work, create, and play.

Work requires movement. Even in our sedentary society, movement is necessary. While working at the computer, you are moving constantly. Keyboarding requires movement of the fingers. You may turn in your seat to check a reference and move your arms, hands, and fingers as you find the specific information you are seeking. You may tap your foot with the music playing in the background. After a few minutes, you need a mental break. You get up and use the muscles of your legs to walk around.

Creativity also incorporates movement. You may think of "creative" people as artists who paint, draw, sing, or play an instrument. All of these activities utilize movement provided by the pull of specific muscles on the appropriate bones. However, "artists" are not the only creative people. Athletes, gardeners, and mechanics are creative, too. Have you ever watched a game of Ultimate Frisbee? The players are constantly adapting to new situations and creating new ways to pass and catch the disc—ways based on what they have practiced, but modified to meet the immediate demands of the situation.

Play utilizes movement. Among children it helps them develop skills needed to function effectively. They learn cooperation, teamwork, and sharing. Their play requires locomotion and manipulation of objects. They move from one place to another as they handle their toys, developing coordination and balance. George Sheehan (1992) believes that once we "find our play" health will take care of itself. "Play maintains our health and promotes our longevity" (p. 298).

Many recognize service toward others as an important aspect of our humanness. Service typically requires movement. Whether you are driving a shut-in to the doctor, building a house with Habitat for Humanity, or working at a food pantry, locomotion is required and so is handling of objects.

Movement gives you the ability to move from place to place. You can enhance your social and intellectual life by meeting people in other places. It allows you to experience new situations. You also must move to obtain the fuel necessary to sustain your life.

Movement requires healthy bones, muscles, ligaments, and tendons. Exercise training develops these structures of motion. Training through regular exercise (see **Box 2.2**) and physical activity gives us greater freedom of movement. A physically healthy person is able to move him- or herself as well as manipulate objects.

Box 2.2 Exercise Recommendations

The American College of Sports Medicine (2006) publishes guidelines for improving health-related physical fitness. They include the following:

- *Cardiorespiratory:* Perform aerobic activities at least 3 days each week for a minimum of 20 minutes at a target heart rate.

- *Muscle strength and endurance:* Perform resistance training at least 2 days per week completing 8–10 exercises using the major muscle groups.

- *Flexibility:* Perform slow, controlled stretching exercises for the major muscle groups 2–3 days per week.

Thought

Thought refers to active use of the mind. The brain is necessary for thought; thus, the brain is the seat of thought (Thomas, 1985). This organ is part of the nervous system, which is the communication center of the body. Thought allows us to adapt, to create, and to move by having new ideas and by transmitting "orders" to the rest of the body. Thought is a prerequisite for most movements. Sheehan (1992) writes that you can train your body and your mind at the same time. Exercise frees the mind to "do whatever it pleases" (p. 173).

Thinking is also known as cognition. This process involves the mental activities that allow you to "create concepts, solve problems, make decisions, and form judgments" (Myers, 2005, p. 358). Creating concepts helps you to organize similar objects (see **Box 2.3**). Your concept of exercise may include jogging, push-ups, and yoga. You can further organize your concepts into hierarchies. You may subdivide exercise into aerobic exercise and resistance exercise. Your concept of aerobic exercise includes activities that utilize large muscle groups, are prolonged, and raise the heart rate. The ability to develop concepts and hierarchies is evidence of thought.

Problem solving is another important component of thought. You learn strategies to help you solve problems. Sometimes you solve problems by trial and error—you keep trying potential solutions until you find one that works. Sometimes you use a step-by-step procedure that guarantees a solution eventually. Imagine that your problem is to find a word that utilizes all of the following letters: XEEEIRSC. You could develop a system that puts each letter into every position until you find a solution. This can be time-consuming if there are many potential solutions. You may also develop simple strategies, called heuristics. In the example above, you can exclude letter combinations with three "Es" in a row, and then begin your trial and error process. Occasionally you have an insight. Perhaps you looked at the letters above and the word "exercise" popped into your head. The inventor of elastic exercise tubing may have had such an experience. Perhaps he was a weight lifter who wanted to train while traveling. He may have been using surgical tubing when he experienced an "ah-ha" moment. The ability to solve problems is another example of effective thought.

You also think when you make decisions and form judgments. Decision making is a higher mental activity using

---

Box 2.3	Which of These Is Not Like the Others?

An old *Sesame Street* activity challenged students to create concepts by asking which of these things is not like the others.

Carrot

Corn

Yogurt

Beans

Broccoli

The seat of thought is
the brain.

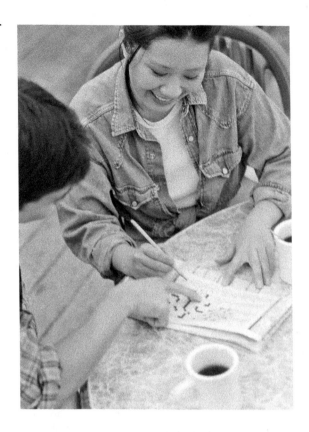

the cortex of the brain. According to Halpern, decision making "involves two or more competing alternatives" (Marzano et al., 1988, p. 48). You make hundreds of decisions every day. You decide whether to skip the French fries or indulge yourself. You make judgments about a friend's trustworthiness as you decide whether to share your problems. For everyday decisions, you usually do not use a complicated process. However, a more systematic approach may be useful for more significant matters.

Decision-making models tend to take a rational approach. Marzano et al. (1988) describe a four-step model that proposes the following: (1) state the goal, (2) generate ideas, (3) prepare a plan, and (4) take action. Decisions are made during each step and these decisions lead naturally to the next phase. A simple example follows. Jason feels fat. His goal is to lose weight, or more specifically, to lose fat. Jason lists possible ways to accomplish this: he could exercise more, watch less television, start a diet, fast, or have liposuction. He evaluates each idea and prepares a plan. Then Jason implements his fat loss plan. Finally, after an appropriate period of time, he evaluates the success of the plan and makes a judgment about its effectiveness.

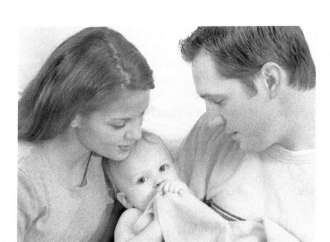

Procreation is the physical capability to continue the species.

Procreation

Procreation is required to sustain the human species. The *Holy Bible* commands humans to "be fruitful and multiply" (Genesis 1:28). Reproduction involves your sexual nature. Sexuality is a complex part of wholeness. Breuss and Richardson (1994) suggest that sexuality has four components: biological, social, psychological, and moral. Entire books have been written on the subject of human sexuality. The focus here is procreation, so the discussion will be limited to the biological component, which includes physiological responses to stimulation, reproduction, puberty, and changes resulting during pregnancy (Breuss & Richardson).

The physical body provides for continuation of the species. Reproduction is a social event. A male and female join together and become one. Males and females each have distinctive reproductive organs that provide the perfect environment for producing the next generation.

Procreation is a distinctive component of physical health because humans are capable of reproduction only during a portion of their lives. Before puberty neither females nor males are capable of reproduction. However, when the sexual organs develop fully during adolescence, reproduction becomes possible. The primary years for producing offspring are the years of young adulthood. Most parents raising children are in this age range. The child-bearing years end for women with menopause. Men, however, can father children into late adulthood.

Continuation of the human species does not require all humans to reproduce. In fact, some choose to avoid sexual contact and others are incapable of reproduction. Still, it is crucial that some humans reproduce in order to sustain the species.

Conclusion

The human body is a marvelous creation. With the cooperation of someone of the opposite gender, it can reproduce. The brain is sometimes referred to as the "master organ." It is capable of thought and controls body function. The body can also move itself from place to place using a variety of means and it can manipulate objects and tools during work and play. The healthy body is wonderful to behold!

Discussion Questions

1. List characteristics of poor physical health.
2. Give examples of how physical health can be related to the other dimensions of health.
3. List three lifestyle changes that would improve your physical health.
4. List specific ways you could build more movement into your daily life.

References

Alters, S., & Schiff, W. (2009). *Essential concepts for healthy living* (5th ed.). Sudbury, MA: Jones and Bartlett.

American College of Sports Medicine. (2006). *ACSM's guidelines for exercise testing and prescription* (7th ed.). Philadelphia: Lippincott Williams & Wilkins.

Balog, J. E. (2005). The meaning of health. *American Journal of School Health, 36*(5), 266–271.

Barnhart, R. K. (Ed.). (1988). *The Barnhart dictionary of etymology.* New York: H. W. Wilson.

Brand, P. & Yancey, P. (1980). *Fearfully and Wonderfully Made.* Grand Rapids MI: Zondervan Publishing House.

Breuss, C. E., & Richardson, G. E. (1994). *Healthy decisions.* Madison, WI: Brown & Benchmark.

Chantrell, C. (Ed.). (2002). *The Oxford dictionary of word histories.* Oxford: Oxford University Press.

Donatelle, R. (2005). *Health: the basics* (6th ed.). San Francisco: Pearson Benjamin Cummings.

Edlin, G., & Golanty, E. (2007). *Health and wellness* (9th ed.). Sudbury, MA: Jones and Bartlett.

Floyd, P. A., Mimms, S. E, & Yelding, C. (2008). *Personal health: perspectives and lifestyles* (4th ed.). Belmont, CA: Thomson Wadsworth.

Foss, M. L., & Keteyian, S. J. (1998). *Fox's physiological basis of exercise and sport* (6th ed.). Boston: WCB McGraw-Hill.

Fox, S. I. (1999). *Human physiology* (6th ed.). Boston: WCB McGraw-Hill.

Gabbard, C. P. (2004). *Lifelong motor development* (4th ed.) San Francisco: Pearson Benjamin Cummings.

Greenberg, J. S. (1985). Health and wellness: a conceptual differentiation. *Journal of School Health, 55*(10), 403–406.

Hales, D. (2009). *An invitation to health.* Belmont, CA: Wadsworth Cengage Learning.

Hyde, J. S. (1994). *Understanding human sexuality* (5th ed.). New York: McGraw-Hill.

Insel, P. M., & Roth, W. T. (2004). *Core concepts in health* (9th ed.). Boston: McGraw-Hill.

Marzano, R. J., Brandt, R. S., Hughes, C. S., Jones, B. F., Presseisen, B. Z., Rankin, S. C., et al. (1988). *Dimensions of thinking: A framework for curriculum and instruction.* Alexandria, VA: Association for Supervision and Curriculum Development.

Myers, D. G. (2005). *Exploring psychology* (6th ed.). New York: Worth.

Ormrod, J. E. (1995). *Human learning* (2nd ed.). Englewood Cliffs, NJ: Merrill.

Payne, V. G., & Isaacs, L. D. (2005). *Human motor development: A lifespan approach* (6th ed.). Boston: McGraw-Hill.

Payne, W. A., & Hahn, D. B. (2002). *Understanding your health* (7th ed.). Boston: McGraw-Hill.

Peck, M. S. (1987). *The different drum: Community making and peace.* New York: Simon & Schuster.

Roizen, M. F. (1999). *Real age: Are you as young as you can be?* New York: Cliff Street.

Sarano, J. (1966). *The meaning of the body* (J. H. Farley, Trans.). Philadelphia: Westminster Press.

Sheehan, G. A. (1992). *Dr. George Sheehan on getting fit and feeling great.* New York: Wings.

Sherwin, B. L. (1991). The human body and the image of God. In D. Cohn-Sherbok (Ed.), *A traditional quest: Essays in honour of Louis Jacobs* (pp. 75–85). Sheffield, England: Sheffield Press.

Thomas, C. L. (Ed.). (1985). *Taber's cyclopedic medical dictionary* (15th ed.). Philadelphia: F.A. Davis.

CHAPTER 3 ▶

Social Health

There is no hope of joy except in human relations.

—Antoine de Saint-Exupery

We must learn to live together as brothers or perish as fools.

—Martin Luther King, Jr.

Introduction

Humans are social creatures who enjoy being with others. Most avoid solitude for fear of loneliness. Studies of institutionalized infants and motherless monkeys demonstrate the importance of bonding at an early age and the detrimental effects when this does not occur (Gardner, 1993). The overlapping nature of the five dimensions of health (physical, social, emotional, intellectual, and spiritual) is apparent when studying social health. The spiritual dimension includes connectedness and the emotional dimension includes relationships. Wisdom, a component of intellectual health, incorporates doing good for others.

The word *social* is derived from two Latin words: *socius* meaning "companion" and *socialis* meaning "united, living together" (Barnhart, 1988; Chantrell, 2002). Several other English words share the same origin: sociable, society, and socialism, for example. From its earliest roots, the word *social* was used in the context of relationships. Social health or wholeness refers to building relationships that enhance well-being.

We all have many types of relationships. We are biologically related to some people, such as our parents, siblings, grandparents, and cousins. We also have work or school relationships. Friends play an important role in most people's lives, and

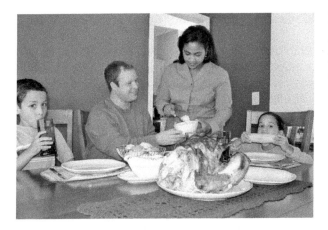

The roots of the word social include living together and companionship.

several types of friendships exist. Acquaintances are people with whom we share particular activities or characteristics, such as teammates on a summer softball team. We even have relationships with strangers. Some believe you can tell a lot about a person by how he or she treats strangers. In fact, one employer likes to dine at a restaurant during job interviews. She believes she can learn much about prospective employees by observing how they interact with the strangers who serve them.

Definitions and Descriptions of Social Health

Payne and Hahn (2002), health educators at Ball State University, suggest that most human development occurs in the presence of others and that this enhances social skills. As people age, their social world expands, and they are exposed to a

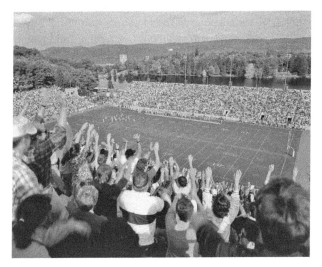

Some relationships are casual. Acquaintances such as fans share interests.

variety of people and social roles. This occurs as they attend new schools, enter the workforce, and travel.

Many types of relationship contribute to social health. Floyd, Mimms, and Yelding (2008), professors at Alabama State University, contend that socially healthy individuals relate well to others, communicate effectively, and respect the needs of others. They also believe that humans have strong needs for acceptance, belonging, and approval.

Health educators Breuss and Richardson (1994) believe that social health includes "good relations with others, the presence of supportive culture, and successful adaptation to the environment" (p. 5).

Insel and Roth (2004) call this dimension "interpersonal and social wellness." They focus on our need for satisfying relationships, suggesting that we need "mutually loving, supportive people in our lives" (p. 3). Communication skills, intimacy, and a support network are all part of social health.

Travis and Ryan (1988) developed a rather complicated model of wellness called the Wellness Energy System. One component of that system is "communicating." This is analogous to the social dimension of health. They suggest that dialogue is crucial for communication; that is, we must listen as well as speak. Characteristics of dialogue include honesty, being fully present in the moment, and nonjudgmental listening. Travis and Ryan also emphasize assertiveness, which is the capacity to clearly and fully state your thoughts and needs while also empathizing with the needs of others.

Donatelle (2005) of Oregon State University suggests that social health includes "your interactions with others on an individual and group basis, your ability to use social resources and support in times of need, and your ability to adapt to a variety of social situations" (p. 33). She points to studies indicating that social health promotes physical health, mental health, and longevity.

Turner, Sizer, Whitney, and Wilks (1992) describe social health as "a state of well-being that results from a person's skill in interacting with other people and with society as a whole" (p. 243). They believe that people who "get along" with others and who have a "social conscience" have the best chance of being socially healthy. Social health requires developing unselfishness, generosity, and a feeling of belonging in society.

Health educator Dianne Hales (2009) writes that

> social health refers to the ability to interact effectively with other people and the social environment, to develop satisfying interpersonal relationships, and to fulfill social roles. It involves participating in and contributing to your community, living in harmony with fellow human beings, developing positive interdependent relationships with others, and practicing healthy sexual behaviors. (p. 6)

Alters and Schiff (2009) suggest that relationships that are "emotionally supportive and intellectually stimulating" will enhance social health. Without social networks, health declines.

These health educators emphasize the value of two-way communication, mutually encouraging relationships, and intimacy.

Models of Social Health

Americans often hold up the strong, silent type as heroes. The cowboy and police officer who work alone and seem to be self-sufficient are examples of this personality type. In reality, people function most effectively in relationships. Several models have been proposed to clarify our social needs.

Interdependence Model

Educator and motivational speaker Stephen Covey (1989) contends that the highest level of human function is not the American ideal of independence. Rather, he believes it is interdependence. Interdependent function is Covey's vision of social health. He proposes three habits that must be developed to achieve interdependent functioning. The three habits or components of social health are (1) think win–win, (2) seek first to understand then to be understood, and (3) synergize.

THINK WIN–WIN

The individual who is able to "think win–win" believes that interpersonal relationships can be of value for all involved. The goal is "mutual benefit" for all parties. Too often people have win–lose philosophies; they believe that in order to get what they want or need, someone else must lose out. Covey describes this as the "scarcity mentality." It is based on competition. Covey subscribes to the "abundance mentality." He believes there is enough to go around—we can all win. This is a paradigm of cooperation. The relationship is "mutually beneficial, mutually satisfying." Under these circumstances all parties feel committed to the relationship.

SEEK FIRST TO UNDERSTAND THEN TO BE UNDERSTOOD

Covey believes that communication is the most important skill in life. We spend many of our waking hours communicating. Unfortunately, much of the time we are either talking or preparing for our next opportunity to talk. We need to listen with the goal of understanding. This is empathic listening. Empathy is the key to developing this habit. Healthful relationships require people to understand each other. By listening first you can discover the other person's needs and desires. Once you understand you can share your own needs and desires.

Empathic listening requires understanding feelings.

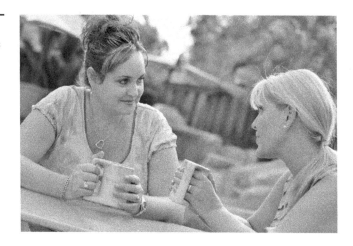

SYNERGIZE

Once you understand each other, you can communicate synergistically. "You are opening your mind and heart and expressions to new possibilities, new alternatives, new options" (Covey, 1989, p. 264). You search for the best solution for any problems or needs. You can function assertively, looking out for both yourself and others. Synergy celebrates diversity, believing that more perspectives provide more potential solutions to problems. You could summarize this component as "two heads are better than one."

Interpersonal Intelligence Model

Psychologist Howard Gardner is a pioneer in the theory of multiple intelligences. He believes that people learn and function in a variety of ways and that different people have different strengths. Interpersonal intelligence is one of the seven types of intelligence he proposed in his book *Frames of Mind* (Gardner, 1993). Gardner identifies four components of interpersonal (social) intelligence: (1) organizing groups, (2) negotiating solutions, (3) personal connection, and (4) social analysis (Goleman, 1995). People with these four skills are natural leaders. They are sought out by peers and co-workers to resolve conflicts. They are invited to parties because they make everyone feel valued and a part of the "in group."

ORGANIZING GROUPS

This refers to a person's ability to coordinate the work of a group of people. Leaders must possess this skill. They identify the needs and skills of others and motivate them to work together toward common goals.

NEGOTIATING SOLUTIONS

This is the special talent of the mediator. Mediators can resolve conflicts and identify win–win solutions. They resolve problems so that everyone feels satisfied. This is not bullying. Bullies resolve problems by force or intimidation. Mediators exhibit empathy and work assertively. They settle arguments and help others work together and get along.

PERSONAL CONNECTION

Empathy helps develop connections between people. Empathic people respond to feelings and concerns. This ability to connect allows people to motivate others, to help a group function smoothly, and to put themselves in the place of another. Empathic people easily develop a rapport with others.

SOCIAL ANALYSIS

The analysts can sense which way the wind is blowing. They recognize "feelings, motives, and concerns" (Goleman, 1995). This recognition allows people to determine a course of action to mobilize others and themselves.

Characteristics of Socially Healthy People

Donatelle (2005) lists several characteristics of socially healthy people. She believes they are able to (1) listen, (2) express themselves, (3) form healthy bonds with others, (4) act in socially acceptable ways, and (5) find a place for themselves in society.

Turner, Sizer, Whitney, and Wilks (1992) suggest that drugs and sexuality play roles in healthy relationships. They write that the socially healthy person: (1) has supportive relationships, (2) has the ability to socialize without the influence of drugs, (3) maintains long-term intimate partnerships, and (4) manages sexual relationships so they improve quality of life.

Turner et al. (1992) also suggest that the basic features of social functioning are communication, cooperation, and compromise. Communication includes both speaking and listening. Cooperation involves working together for the good of all, and compromise is a willingness to give up something you want so others can get something they want.

Psychologist Joel Block (1980) studied friendship. He believes that humans long for friendship and identifies three "nutrients" that nourish friendship: authenticity, acceptance, and direct expression. These might be considered characteristics of social health. *Authenticity* refers to being genuine. Many people are afraid to show what they are really like—they fear people won't like them if they see the

Cooperation and helping others builds relationships.

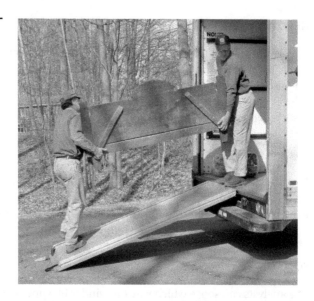

real person. Authentic friends are more spontaneous and less calculating. They have enough self-confidence to be themselves. *Acceptance* is respect for the individuality of others. There is no pressure to be something or someone else. When you are accepting of others, they know they will not be judged by you for being different or weak or frightened. Finally, *direct expression* is the ability to communicate what you need and feel. Direct expression takes the mystery out of communication. In my own family we have a saying, "I still can't read your mind." We say this in response to indirect communication and when we feel messages have been unclear. Finally, direct expression is the ability to communicate what you need and feel (see **Box 3.1**).

Health writer Florence Isaacs (1999) suggests several "rules" for friendship and social health.

1. Don't betray a confidence. Healthy relationships require trust.
2. Reciprocate. Relationships require effort from all parties. If one person does all the work, he or she will eventually feel unappreciated. Affirmation of the friend is also part of reciprocation.
3. Spend time together. Rituals can help achieve this. If distance prevents you from seeing each other, use the phone to maintain the relationship.
4. Avoid criticism and intrusion. Constant judgment weakens a relationship.

Box 3.1 Communication Styles

Kim asks Chris if he would like to go to a movie. He could answer in many ways. Which of the following is direct?

• We could do that.
• I heard that it's a good movie.
• Yes, let's go tonight.
• That's an interesting idea.
• I like comedies.

Acceptance strengthens it. Give friends the opportunity to develop other relationships as well.

5. Celebrate others' success. Unhealthy relationships may include envy. Healthy friendships want the best for the other. A true friend enjoys your good grades as much as you do.

Healthy relationships are characterized by effective communication and by nourishment. High levels of social health enhance your sense of well-being. The socially healthy individual is concerned with both him- or herself and others.

A New Model of Social Health

Social health occurs in the context of supportive relationships, the potential to adapt to new variables within relationships, and the recognition of our interdependence with those around us. Within that context, effective communication (dialogue) is the foundation of social health. Concern for the well-being of others (empathy) is the basis for health-enhancing relationships. The deepest relationships are characterized by intimacy. Not all relationships reach this level. **Figure 3.1** illustrates this model of social health.

Context

Social health does not occur in a vacuum. There are prerequisites. We might think of these variables as the rich soil in which social health can grow and develop. Supportive relationships provide freedom to be honest, to disagree, and to change. Interdependence recognizes that no one is an island. Virtually everything we do depends on others. In general, we do not grow our own food, build our own cars or houses, or educate ourselves. We need others for these activities. Adaptability involves our ability to grow and develop. We change as we age and learn, and we must recognize that others do the same. Adaptability means that relationships can persist even as they change.

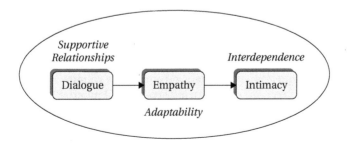

Figure 3.1 A Model of Social Health

Dialogue

Dialogue emphasizes that communication is two-directional. Information is sent and received by all parties. Dialogue requires self-disclosure, listening, and feedback (Insel & Roth, 2004). First, we must be willing to reveal information about ourselves—what we like and dislike, what we feel, and what we want or need. We need to be clear and direct. "I" statements are usually more effective because they avoid blame and accusatory tones, which often cause others to stop listening. Consider the following attempts at communication: "You are so inconsiderate. You are never on time." In this case, the listener is likely to feel attacked and may become defensive. An alternative would be, "I feel disappointed and unappreciated when you are late for our dates." The second statement is an "I" statement. It focuses on the speaker's feelings. The listener can respond to the speaker's feelings rather than trying to defend himself.

Listening is a difficult skill. Few of us are skilled listeners. Too often we spend our "listening" time preparing a response. We are not fully engaged in what the speaker is communicating. Effective listeners don't interrupt, but they do provide appropriate nonverbal feedback such as making eye contact or nodding. They also respect the speaker and are able to communicate their interest in what he or she is trying to say.

Finally, we must provide feedback to be sure the message sent is the message received. The roles are reversed and the listener becomes a speaker to ensure he or she understands the original message. A barrier to effective dialogue occurs when there are misunderstandings. Feedback allows clarification of the message and corrections if necessary.

Empathy

The kind of exchange described in the previous section leads naturally into empathy. Empathy is the "ability to put oneself in the place of other people and appreciate their feelings" (Karren, Hafen, Smith, & Frandsen, 2002, p. 558). Stephen Covey (1989) labels the kind of listening described above as empathic listening. It requires listening for meaning, not just information. It connects people and forms a "glue" between them (Karren et al.). Feeling empathy moves us from self-concern to concern for the well-being of others. When others feel cared for, relationships are strengthened.

Researcher Allan Luks (1991) has studied volunteerism. He distinguishes between empathy and sympathy. When you emphasize your own feelings about another's situation, you are experiencing sympathy. Empathy is "discovering inside yourself how these problems feel to the other person" (p. 193).

Intimacy

The word *intimacy* has become associated with sexual activity. If someone asks, "Were you intimate?" they might be asking if you had sexual intercourse.

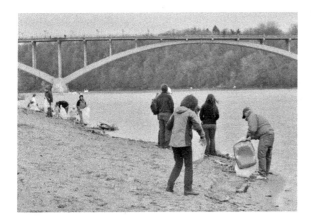

Working together towards a common goal can improve social health.

This is a very narrow view of intimacy. Two broader characteristics of intimacy are sharing and trust. Both parties feel safe sharing their thoughts, feelings, beliefs, fears, and goals. Each person knows they will be loved and appreciated even if the other disagrees with them.

Most of us seek intimacy, but it is a rare occurrence. It is possible in a relationship only when we trust another enough to share all our thoughts and feelings (Thomas & Kotecki, 2007). We seek it because many needs can be fulfilled in intimate relationships: "the need for approval and affirmation, for companionship, for meaningful ties and a sense of belonging, for sexual satisfaction" (Insel & Roth, 2004, p. 90). Some of these needs can be fulfilled in more superficial relationships as well. But intimate relationships are the deepest, most rewarding, and most durable. Many people seek intimacy in marriage, but friendships and family relationships can be intimate as well.

Rebecca Donatelle (2005) writes that intimate relationships are characterized by four components: (1) behavioral interdependence, (2) need fulfillment, (3) emotional attachment, and (4) emotional availability. *Behavioral interdependence* refers to the fact that people have a "mutual impact" on each other. The actions, thoughts, and opinions of one affect the other. Relationships can also fulfill psychological *needs* to share desires, feelings, and fears; to nurture others and assist them in times of need; and to be assured of our own value. *Emotional attachment* refers to the love felt in intimate relationships. We may need to think of love broadly and without a sexual component to fully appreciate this characteristic. *Emotional availability* is the ability to give and receive without fear of rejection or ridicule.

Conclusion

Humans are social beings. We seek a sense of belonging and of being valued through our relationships. We experience social health when our relationships contribute to our well-being. In order for this to happen we must learn to communicate effectively. This requires both listening and speaking skills. The best listeners are empathic. They are able to "get inside" others and really understand them. The healthiest relationships are characterized by intimacy. Intimate relationships may occur between spouses, family members, and friends. They are trusting relationships in which both parties trust each other enough to share their deepest thoughts and feelings.

Discussion Questions

1. List examples of relationships. Which are most crucial for social health?
2. Compare and contrast the interdependence (Covey) and interpersonal intelligence (Gardner) models of social health.
3. Describe a time when you felt someone was particularly empathic while listening to you.
4. What are the characteristics of intimate relationships?

References

Alters, S., & Schiff, W. (2009). *Essential concepts for healthy living* (5th ed.). Sudbury, MA: Jones and Bartlett.

Barnhart, R. K. (ed.). (1988). *The Barnhart dictionary of etymology*. New York: H.W. Wilson.

Block, J. D. (1980). *Friendship: How to give it, how to get it*. New York: Macmillan.

Breuss, C. E., & Richardson, G. E. (1994). *Healthy decisions*. Madison, WI: Brown & Benchmark.

Chantrell, C. (ed.). (2002). *The Oxford dictionary of word histories*. Oxford: Oxford University Press.

Covey, S. R. (1989). *The 7 habits of highly effective people*. New York: Simon & Schuster.

Donatelle, R. (2005). *Health: The basics* (6th ed.). San Francisco: Pearson Benjamin Cummings.

Floyd, P. A., Mimms, S. E., & Yelding, C. (2008). *Personal health: Perspectives and lifestyles* (4th ed.). Belmont, CA: Thomson Wadsworth.

Gardner, H. (1993). *Frames of mind: The theory of multiple intelligences*. New York: Basic.

Goleman, D. (1995). *Emotional intelligence: Why it can matter more than IQ*. New York: Bantam.

Hales, D. (2009). *An invitation to health*. Belmont, CA: Wadsworth Cengage Learning.

Insel, P. M., & Roth, W. T. (2004). *Core concepts in health* (9th ed.). Boston: McGraw-Hill.

Isaacs, F. (1999). *Toxic friends, true friends*. New York: William Morrow.

Karren, K. J., Hafen, B. Q., Smith, N. L., & Frandsen, K. J. (2002). *Mind/body health: The effects of attitudes, emotions, and relationships* (2nd ed.). San Francisco: Benjamin Cummings.

Luks, A. (1991). *The healing power of doing good: The health and spiritual benefits of helping others*. New York: Fawcett Columbine.

Payne, W. A., & Hahn, D. B. (2002). *Understanding your health* (7th ed.). Boston: McGraw-Hill.

Thomas, D. Q., & Kotecki, J. E.(2007). *Physical activity and health: An interactive approach* (2nd ed.). Sudbury, MA: Jones and Bartlett.

Travis, J. W., & Ryan, R. S. (1988). *Wellness workbook* (2nd ed.). Berkeley, CA: Ten Speed Press.

Turner, L. W., Sizer, F. S., Whitney, E. N., & Wilks, B. B. (1992). *Life choices: Health concepts and strategies* (2nd ed.) St. Paul, MN: West.

CHAPTER 4 ▶

Emotional Health

Anyone can become angry—that is easy. But to be angry with the right person, to the right degree, at the right time, for the right purpose, and in the right way—this is not easy.

—Aristotle

The goal is balance, not emotional suppression: every feeling has its value and significance.

—Daniel Goleman, 1995

Introduction

"He makes me so mad!" "I couldn't help myself!" "I'm just the jealous type!" "I love my dog." These statements all contain feelings or what psychologists call emotions. But they don't provide much information about our emotions or how we can recognize and develop emotional health. The goal of this chapter is to provide insights into emotional health.

The Latin word *movere* means "to move" and the prefix *e-* means "out" (Chantrell, 2002). The English word *emotion* came into usage during the sixteenth century and meant "a sense of strong feeling, mental agitation" (Barnhart, 1988, p. 326). More current definitions of emotion include "instinctive feelings such as pity, hate, love" (Chantrell, p. 174) and "any strong manifestation or disturbance of the conscious or the unconscious mind, typically involuntary and often leading to complex bodily changes and forms of behavior" (*Funk & Wagnalls*, 1989, p. 414).

Health writers Turner, Sizer, Whitney, and Wilks (1992) define an emotion as "a felt tendency to move toward something assessed as good or favorable or away from something assessed as bad or unfavorable" (p. 35). It is interesting that they have incorporated the original Latin meaning of movement into their definition.

Psychologists and educators often refer to the affective domain of learning. Affective can be defined as "pertaining to or arising from feeling or emotional reactions rather than from thought" (*Funk & Wagnalls*, 1989, p. 24). Thus, affect is distinguished from the intellectual or cognitive aspects of human functioning.

Erika Hunter is a social worker and psychologist who wrote a book titled *Little Book of Big Emotions* (Hunter, 2004). She describes emotions as energy. This energy can be either used or misused. Emotional health refers to productive use of emotions. Hunter proposes five basic emotions—anger, sorrow, shame, fear, and gladness. *Anger* has several variables. It can push you toward new ideas, growth, and change, or it can lead to violence and addiction. Anger can be directed inward toward yourself or outward at others. For example, anger about a poor exam score can be directed inward and motivate us to change our study habits. This would be healthy; however, your anger could also be directed at the instructor and result in a verbal attack against him. This is obviously unproductive. *Sorrow* occurs when we lose something, whether it is big or small, concrete or abstract. Sorrow is a very personal experience that often leads to loneliness. Whether your pet grasshopper dies or your parents divorce, you feel loss. Hunter defines *shame* as "feeling bad about something that is not our fault" (p. 22). This differs from guilt, which occurs when someone feels bad about something that is his or her fault. During the 1998 Olympic ice dancing competition one pair fell when the male lost his balance. You can be sure that both skaters felt bad about the fall. The male was at fault; he lost his balance. The emotion he felt was guilt. The female also felt bad, even though she was not to blame for the fall. She experienced shame. *Fear* often results in an urge either to run away or to fight. Both options clearly require energy. When your safety is threatened, you feel fear. Fear often seems to hijack the rational part of the brain and you experience impulses to act, to protect yourself. *Gladness* signifies a "contented heart." There is a sense of living in the moment and of gratitude.

There is some debate about how many emotions exist. Ekman (2003) proposes "families" of basic emotions, and this leads to disagreement about the number of distinct emotions. He would argue that there are multiple expressions or types of anger, for example. An angry person may be furious, enraged, frustrated, or dismayed. Others would say that each of these is a separate emotion.

Daniel Goleman (1995) suggests that there are "hundreds of emotions, along with their blends, variations, mutations, and nuances" (p. 289). However, he proceeds to propose eight likely possibilities as the basic or fundamental emotions: anger, sadness, fear, enjoyment, love, surprise, disgust, and shame. Each basic emotion has family members or what you might think of as subemotions.

Psychologist Carroll Izard (Myers, 2001) studied facial expressions of infants to determine how many emotions were present at birth. She identified 10 basic emotions—joy, interest-excitement, surprise, sadness, anger, disgust, contempt,

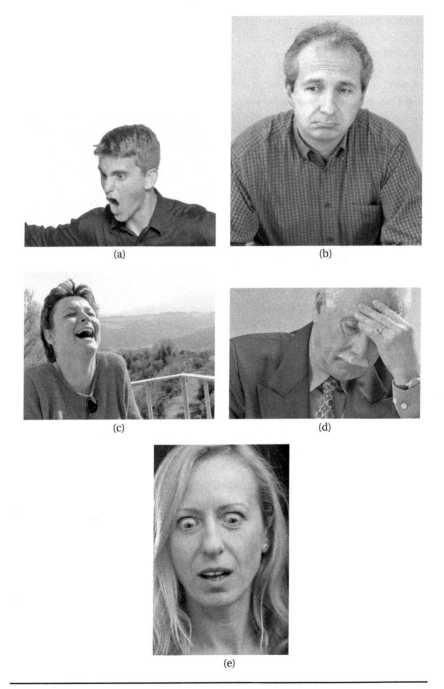

(a)

(b)

(c)

(d)

(e)

Healthy people experience a variety of emotions: (a) Anger, (b) Sadness, (c) Joy, (d) Guilt, and (e) Fear.

fear, shame, and guilt. She believes that other "emotions" are simply combinations of these. For example, love (which most of us would identify as a basic emotion) is a mixture of joy and interest-excitement.

Emotions are part of daily life. We experience a range of emotions every day, but these emotions affect each of us differently. They contribute to our humanness and are a component of who we are. Health is the well-being of the whole person, and our emotions are part of that whole. Psychologist Claude Steiner (1997) believes each of us can become "emotional gourmets." We can become "aware of the texture, flavor, and aftertaste of [our] emotions" (p. 12).

Definitions and Descriptions of Emotional Health

Psychologists Peter Salovey and John Mayer (1990) use the phrase *emotional intelligence* to describe emotional health. They suggest that emotional intelligence involves the "ability to monitor one's own and others' feelings and emotions, to discriminate among them and to use this information to guide one's thinking and actions" (p. 189).

Daniel Goleman (1998) builds on the work of Salovey and Mayer in his book titled *Emotional Intelligence*. He defines emotional intelligence as "the capacity for recognizing our own feelings and those of others, for motivating ourselves, and for managing emotions well in ourselves and in our relationships" (p. 317). He believes that intellectual and emotional intelligence complement each other and provide for synergy. Synergy occurs when the whole is greater than the sum of its parts. We function at a higher level when we utilize both intellectual and emotional capacities.

Emotional health is often linked to our ability to manage stress. Payne and Hahn (2002) of Ball State University suggest that emotional health includes our "ability to cope with stress, remain flexible, and compromise to resolve conflict" (p. 18). We often suggest exercise (physical), meditation (spiritual), or "talking it out" (social) to keep stress from overwhelming us.

Some authors focus on behavior. Breuss and Richardson (1994) define emotional health as the "ability to express emotions comfortably and appropriately" (p. 5). This implies that sometimes we would not express our emotions at all. It is interesting that both "comfortably" and "appropriately" are included. There may be times when we would feel comfortable expressing an emotion, but it would not be appropriate. Perhaps you are meeting your boy- or girlfriend's parents for the first time. Their lack of concern over protecting the environment angers you. If you want to improve the chance of this relationship continuing, it would not be appropriate to express your anger. You may have a chance to debate the issue at another time.

Dealing with the changes that occur throughout life is the focus of Floyd, Mimms, and Yelding (2003). They suggest that the emotionally healthy are "able

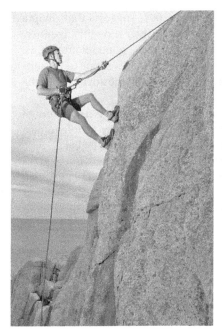 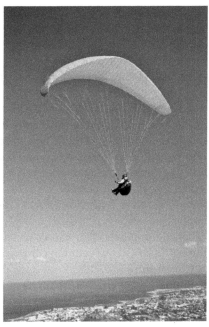

Overcoming challenges can improve emotional health.

to adjust to change, face challenges and problems, and enjoy life" (p. 2). There is an element of flexibility in their lives. For example, imagine that you have planned a spring break trip to Florida. After driving through the night, you arrive at the beach in Florida. You step out of your van and discover the beach is closed due to high pollution levels. This requires a change in plan. You must face the challenge. An emotionally healthy response would be to get back in the van and drive to a new camping area. An unhealthy response would be to get angry (at whom?), sulk, and suffer through the week without any time at the beach.

Emotional health is closely related to physical and social health. Psychologist David Myers (2001) refers to the relationship between physical and emotional health as "embodied emotion." Physiological changes accompany emotions. If a dog jumps out at you in the dark, your muscles tense, heart rate increases, and sugar is released into the bloodstream. Turner et al. (1992) suggest that emotionally healthy people take care of their bodies, but that emotionally unhealthy individuals are prone to drug abuse, heart disease, and cancer. They also believe that the emotionally healthy relate well to themselves, to others, and to society as a whole. Emotionally healthy people have intimate friends with whom they can discuss their problems.

The American Academy of Family Physicians (2002) suggests that people are emotionally healthy when they are "in control of their thoughts, feelings, and behaviors. They feel good about themselves and have good relationships. They can keep their problems in perspective." The themes seem to be self-control, relationships that improve one's life, self-esteem, and the ability to see the big picture.

Edlin and Golanty (2007) also believe that stress management is a component of social health. In addition, they write that emotionally healthy people understand their emotions and know how to cope with problems of daily living.

Seaward (2001) defines emotional health as "the ability to feel and express the entire range of human emotions and to control them, not be controlled by them" (p. 19). This perspective values all emotions, implying that each has a place in our lives. It also implies that we can choose how we will deal with our emotions.

These descriptions of emotional health provide some insight. Behavior, which is the expression of our emotions, is an important indicator of emotional health. Our relationships with others also provide information about emotional health. Adaptation is also crucial. We all have to deal with changes in our lives. The emotionally healthy person can do that more easily.

Models of Emotional Health

Our emotions and how to live productively with them have been popular topics of study. Psychologists have defined, identified, and categorized emotions. They have also developed models that help us understand emotional health. Three models are summarized in this section.

Emotional Intelligence Model (Salovey)

Salovey and Mayer (1990), psychologists at Yale University and University of New Hampshire, respectively, propose a model of emotional intelligence that includes three components: (1) appraisal and expression of emotion, (2) regulation of emotion, and (3) utilization of emotion. An examination of each component will help increase your understanding of emotional health.

APPRAISAL AND EXPRESSION OF EMOTION

We perform this action both internally and externally; that is, we appraise and express our own emotions (internal) and those of others (external). Internally, emotional health can be assessed and expressed both verbally and nonverbally. We must be able to speak clearly about our emotions. People who are unable to

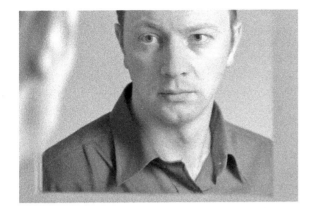

Looking at yourself in a mirror may help you recognize the emotion you are feeling.

appraise and express their emotions are referred to as alexithymic. Alexithymics exhibit poor emotional health.

You can learn to recognize signs of happiness or anger. Perhaps a chance look in the mirror will tell you why friends are avoiding you—is that anger they see? Or maybe you get headaches when you feel jealous. People who are emotionally healthy can process internal emotional information, quickly recognize what they are feeling, and respond to their own emotions.

Emotionally healthy people can perform the same functions with others. Recognizing what others are feeling may enhance interpersonal cooperation. If you can recognize when someone is unhappy or angry, you can respond to that emotion in a way that will maintain or strengthen the relationship. Appraisal and expression of emotion often occurs nonverbally. For example, facial expressions are quite predictable across cultures. Psychologist Paul Ekman (2003) has found that people can recognize happiness and anger in virtually any culture.

The ability to accurately appraise another's emotions can contribute to empathy. Empathy is more than just recognition—it also includes the ability to experience another's feelings. Salovey and Mayer (1990) believe that empathy is a crucial characteristic of emotionally healthy behavior. Empathy increases the likelihood that advice you offer will be accepted as valuable. Empathy motivates altruistic behavior. Empathic people are able to understand the point of view of others, to identify the emotions of others, to experience appropriate emotions in response to others, and to communicate this internal experience to others. When Coach Roy Williams won his first national collegiate basketball championship in 2005, his first thought was for the losing coach (Feinstein, 2006). Coach Williams had lost in the title game previously, and he knew how it felt. He immediately sought out Coach Weber of the University of Illinois to console him. Then Coach Williams began his celebration. That is empathy.

REGULATION OF EMOTION

The second component of the Salovey and Mayer (1990) model is regulation. They suggest that most of the research in this area has focused on moods, which are described as "less intense and generally longer lasting than emotions" (p. 196). Nonetheless, they feel that research on moods can inform the discussion of emotional intelligence. Regulation of emotion has two components: regulation in oneself and regulation in others. Self-regulation can be achieved in several ways. For example, if listening to rock music makes you happy, you can seek the experience of listening to that music again. You can help bring about those feelings of happiness. Similarly, if scary movies give you nightmares, you could avoid them. Thus, your behaviors and experiences affect your emotions. You can also regulate your emotions by choosing your associates. If you always feel valued and loved when spending time with your siblings, schedule time and activities with them. If you find yourself feeling stupid and worthless when you spend time with your roommate, perhaps you should find a new roommate. Seek out people who help you maintain a positive view of yourself.

Emotional health also includes the ability to regulate the emotions of others. Effective speakers can alter the mood of an audience. They can provide rewarding experiences for their listeners. A supportive friend or associate may help others feel good about themselves. The emotionally healthy person may plan activities for friends or families. They focus on what makes others happy. They can reinforce positive self-assessments of others when they are with them or may be able to help diffuse a friend's anger. It is important to note that these behaviors could also be used in manipulative ways to gain control over others. The emotionally healthy person influences others to worthwhile ends.

UTILIZATION OF EMOTION

This brings us to the third component of emotional intelligence. Emotionally healthy people can utilize the energy of their emotions to solve problems and live productively. Emotions can produce conditions that allow new levels of problem solving. For example, emotions may cause stress. When people experience stress, hormones are released. These hormones increase energy and improve brain function. Therefore, we can understand that it is normal and beneficial to be nervous before an important test.

Emotional Intelligence Model (Goleman)

Psychologist Daniel Goleman (1995) expanded the Salovey and Mayer (1990) model to five components, adding an interpersonal perspective. The five components are: (1) knowing your emotions, (2) managing your emotions, (3) motivating yourself, (4) empathy, and (5) handling relationships.

KNOWING YOUR EMOTIONS

Knowing your emotions is a type of mindfulness, a true awareness of what is happening inside you at a particular moment. You may question the significance of this, thinking "I know when I am jealous." In reality, you may not recognize your jealousy until later. Looking back, you may say, "I thought I was just angry. I didn't realize how jealous I really was." This self-awareness by itself is a neutral event. It may simply be naming the emotion while you are experiencing it. It may mean stepping back from the experience for a moment to evaluate it. You are aware of both your emotion and your thoughts about it. This analysis has an intellectual component as you evaluate what you are feeling.

MANAGING YOUR EMOTIONS

Goleman relates managing your emotions to the virtue of temperance. Neither suppressing the emotion nor losing control of yourself is productive. Temperance seeks a balance between these two. Extremes "undermine our stability" (p. 56). Management allows you to soothe yourself and to terminate an emotion or mood. The ability to manage your emotions allows you to recover quickly from events and pressures.

MOTIVATING YOURSELF

Achieving goals requires several capacities. Perhaps foundational is the capacity to control impulses and delay gratification. Emotions lead you to act—impulse control allows you to wait. If you really want to get fit, you must control the impulse to quit your workout early. The goal is more important than short-term gratification. Optimism is another tool for motivating yourself. It reflects hope for the future. Optimism protects against apathy, depression, and hopelessness. Finally, flow contributes to motivation. Flow is a state in which you are so consumed by your activity that you lose track of time and surroundings. Athletes often refer to flow as being "in the zone." Finding and participating in activities that produce flow is also motivating. Emotionally intelligent (or healthy) people motivate themselves by their optimistic orientation and by finding flow. They control their impulses in order to achieve longer term goals.

EMPATHY

Emotional health impacts us socially. Recognizing the emotions the people around you are feeling is a crucial people skill. When conversing, empathic people not only hear the content of the conversation, but also recognize the underlying feelings. They are able to "put themselves in the other's shoes." Self-aware people are better at understanding the emotions of others. Empathy obviously enhances social health as well. Empathic people identify with those around them. It is more than sympathy—empathy joins with others in their feelings.

HANDLING RELATIONSHIPS

Social competence involves managing emotions in others. You send "emotional signals" during every interaction. Your emotions affect those you are with, and their emotions affect you. Those who forcefully express feelings can transfer their emotions to the more passive person. Emotionally intelligent people are able to make us feel good. We are "infected" by them. Those with high levels of social intelligence interact with others easily and connect with them. They are not simply "social chameleons." Social chameleons are experts at making a good first impression. They will say anything for social approval. This does not encourage healthy relationships. The truly healthy person is aware of the needs and desires of both parties. There is integrity between the public and private personas. Socially competent people are genuine and trustworthy.

Emotional Energy Model

Hunter (2004) proposes a three-component model of emotional health. First we must experience our emotions. Hunter believes that some people resist or deny their emotions, which is unhealthy. Instead we must be aware of our emotions. Second, she recommends that we name the emotions and learn to distinguish one from another. This leads to the third step—we must choose whether to act on our emotions. The statements at the beginning of this chapter imply that we do not have that choice. Hunter suggests that although we cannot choose whether to *have* an emotion, we can decide what to *do* with it. She writes that "when we release their [emotions'] energy in healthy ways, we gain important information that leads to understanding and maturity" (p. 18).

It is clear from these models that emotions can either enhance or impair health. Ignoring or suppressing emotions results in poor health. In contrast, recognizing and managing emotions helps us to live full lives.

Characteristics of Emotionally Healthy People

Payne and Hahn (2002) believe that emotional health is reflected in your response to changes in your environment. "Emotionally healthy people feel good about their responses to change, whereas those who are negative about their own feelings and their responses to changes are less emotionally healthy" (p. 30). They also suggest that emotionally healthy people feel comfortable with themselves, experience the full range of emotions, are not overwhelmed by their emotions, receive and give love easily, and feel concern for others.

Insel and Roth (2004) list several characteristics of emotional health. They believe that emotionally healthy people are optimistic and trusting. They also have high self-esteem, self-confidence, and self-control. Their relationships are "satisfying." Finally, they are able to share their feelings. Thomas and Kotecki (2007) agree with these characteristics and add that emotionally healthy people feel "capable, courageous, worthy, respected, appreciated, and loved" (p. 7).

Turner et al. (1992) believe that we must keep growing and deal with life changes to develop emotional health. They propose a long list of characteristics of the emotionally healthy (p. 40):

1. High self-esteem
2. Confident that their behavior is normal
3. Honest
4. Accept themselves
5. Can have fun
6. Don't take themselves too seriously
7. Can have intimate relationships
8. Do not manipulate others
9. Take responsibility appropriately
10. Are able to grieve
11. Live with balance

Psychologists often use the term *happiness* or the phrase *subjective well-being* in contexts related to emotional health. Psychologist David Myers (2001) lists several factors related to happiness. He suggests that happy people tend to have high self-esteem, close friendships or a satisfying marriage, work and leisure activities that engage their skills, and meaningful religious faith. They also tend to be optimistic, sleep well, and exercise regularly.

A New Model of Emotional Health

Emotions provide instant plans for action (Goleman, 1995). Emotionally healthy individuals recognize emotions as they occur. They feel free to experience the emotion, and they are able to monitor and control their behavioral response. Sometimes emotions should be expressed. At other times they should be suppressed, at least temporarily. This leads us to a simple model of emotional health (see **Figure 4.1**).

Mindfulness (of Your Emotions)

Mindfulness is often associated with spiritual health (Donatelle, 2006; Scandurra, 1999), but it also relates to the emotional component. Mindfulness can be described as "awareness and acceptance of the reality of the present moment"

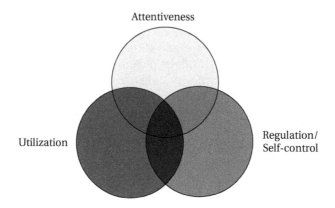

Attentiveness

Utilization

Regulation/
Self-control

Figure 4.1 A Model of Emotional Health

(Donatelle, p. 45). Mindfulness is related to the concepts of appraisal (Salovey and Mayer, 1990) and knowing (Goleman, 1995), which are described earlier in this chapter; however, mindfulness implies a deeper awareness. We not only recognize the emotion we are feeling, but also focus on it. We may analyze it by asking questions. **Box 4.1** poses questions suggested by Scandurra. Thinking about emotions we experience helps us understand their roots.

At a fundamental level, mindfulness means we can distinguish between different emotions. We can recognize the difference between anger and jealousy, for example. It also means we recognize that we can experience emotions at different intensities. Finally, it helps us develop a vocabulary to talk about our feelings.

Mindfulness also incorporates causality. You recognize the roots of your emotions, as well as your emotional tendencies—what makes you happy, mad, or anxious. You discover your emotional triggers and your typical response to them. Some people experience anxiety when they feel unprepared. Knowing this and being aware of triggers such as deadlines can help you control the anxiety. You may even be able to prevent or reduce it by preparing early for exams or papers. Awareness and appraisal of your emotional state enhances your ability to control how you express these emotions.

If you can't recognize what you are feeling, the emotion can overwhelm you. Goleman (1995) calls the ability to recognize your emotions *self-awareness*

Box 4.1 Enhancing Mindfulness of Anger

Where in the body is the anger?

Does the body become hard or soft with anger?

Are different kinds of anger present?

How does the anger affect breathing?

How does the anger affect perceptions of pain?

How does the anger affect my thinking?

and describes it as the foundation of emotional health. The emotionally healthy person is able to verbalize what is being felt.

Another aspect of mindfulness is the ability to recognize what others are feeling. This builds empathy, which Goleman (1995) calls the fundamental people skill. Steiner (1997) suggests that empathy may be a sixth sense. Some psychologists believe that "empaths" perceive emotional information in the same way that the eyes perceive visual stimuli. Empathic individuals are attuned to the wants and needs of others. This ability allows them to work well with and care for those around them.

Experiencing the Spectrum of Emotions

Experts disagree about the number of emotions. Hunter (2004) suggests there are only five, whereas Goleman (1995) identifies eight. It is clear that a spectrum of emotions exist. Some emotions serve to attract us toward some phenomenon or person; for example, feeling love toward someone motivates us to spend time with him or her. Other emotions repel—they cause us to distance ourselves from the situation; for example, the sound of rustling leaves while walking in the dark causes fear and our response is to run.

Emotions, then, serve a purpose. Different emotions motivate us to accomplish different things. To identify some emotions as negative and others as positive is to misunderstand emotions. Goleman's (1995) description of emotions as "instant plans for action" helps us recognize this. We should acknowledge the potential value of all emotions.

Cultural traditions may contradict this idea. For example, in some ethnic groups men are expected to be strong and brave. To cry or show fear demonstrates weakness. However, the healthy man understands that sadness is sometimes appropriate and that showing that sadness is also appropriate. The death of a loved one would certainly be an example of a time to show sadness.

Women are sometimes maligned for showing anger. They are expected to quietly bear with it. However, holding anger in is unproductive. Eventually a minor inconvenience may result in an eruption. That eruption may be directed at the wrong person.

The variety of emotions makes life more interesting. In Caroline Knapp's (1996) autobiography, *Drinking: A Love Story*, she describes an Alcoholics Anonymous meeting. Knapp relates the story of a young woman early in sobriety who recalled that while she was drinking she had only two emotions, anxiety and despair. The woman goes on to say, "'Now I have, like, too many to count and . . . some of them are really, really good'" (Knapp, p. 247). During recovery this woman's health was improving, and one indicator of that was experiencing a wider range of emotions.

Health relates to the whole person. Emotional health relates to the entire spectrum of emotions. Emotionally healthy people experience a smorgasbord of feelings. None are "good" or "bad." All can help us live fully. However, it is important to control our impulses to act so that emotions enhance our health.

Regulation and Self-Control of Your Emotions

The physiological responses to each emotion are predictable and useful (Goleman, 1995). For example, anger results in increased blood flow to the hands, making it easier to grasp a weapon. Heart rate increases and adrenaline is released, providing energy for action such as fight or flight. In contrast, when you are happy, brain activity inhibits negative feelings and worries. This provides a period of rest. The rested individual is ready for and enthusiastic about the next task. Emotions are experienced.

Erika Hunter (2004) distinguishes between *having* emotions and *indulging* in them. Suppressing emotions is unnatural. Holding back is a temporary solution. Eventually the emotions rush out, and when that happens, some people become physically or verbally abusive. Even though emotions are experienced, we do have the ability to regulate our responses. The goal is to express and act on our emotions without harming others. This requires mindfulness and regulation. We can take charge of our emotions.

Some emotional triggers are learned. Connections between the triggers and emotional responses are established in the brain. These connections seem to be "permanent physiological records of what we have learned" (Ekman, 2003). We cannot unlearn the trigger but we can learn to interrupt it. For example, we may rehearse situations that are emotional triggers to become accustomed to them. Thus, the emotional response is weakened. Imagine that when you were teased by classmates as a young child, you felt humiliated and angry. An emotional response to teasing has been learned. As an adult, you can weaken this by evaluating episodes of teasing. You can identify the motivation for teasing and realize that the goal is not to humiliate you. You can anticipate teasing and brace yourself for it so that you do not interpret it as humiliating. As a result, you may be better able to control your temper.

Do not fight your emotions. The goal is not to shut them off, but to experience them and respond appropriately. People who don't show their emotions are often perceived as unfeeling, detached, or even inhuman (Ekman, 2003). To learn from your emotions, you must experience them. As you do this, you will find that you can recognize them more easily. Emotionally healthy people experience the full range of emotions. They are able to regulate them and have learned how to end an emotion if it is unproductive. They can also minimize emotional behavior they would regret later, subdue emotional expressions, and avoid harmful actions or words.

Emotions provide energy for action. They are empowering (Steiner, 1997) if you learn to let them work for you rather than against you. They can be rewarding if you learn to express them productively, which leads us to the fourth component of emotional health: utilization.

Utilization of Your Emotions

The emotionally healthy individual is "able to handle emotions in a way that improves your personal power and improves the quality of life around you" (Steiner, 1997, p. 11). Emotional health "improves relationships, creates loving possibilities between people, makes cooperative work possible, and facilitates the feeling of community" (Steiner, p. 11).

As mentioned earlier, anger causes increased heart rate and blood flow, as well as a rush of hormones such as adrenaline. Thus, more energy is available for action. The traditional actions are fight or flight. However, fight and flight are inappropriate actions for most causes of our anger. For example, imagine that you are sitting down for a history exam. You read the first question and realize that the class did not discuss the topic. When you read the second question, you feel the professor has picked an obscure portion of the readings. At this point, you feel the exam is unfair, and you become angry at the professor. Neither running from the room nor hitting the professor is an appropriate response for your anger. The question becomes, "How can I use this energy to resolve the problem?" Perhaps you can use your heightened senses to remember something about the reading you did, or maybe you can use the extra blood flowing to the brain to brainstorm potential ways to answer the questions.

Interactivity is another way to use emotions. Steiner (1997) believes this is a sophisticated level of utilization. Emotions combine within and between people. Interactive people recognize and predict this. This knowledge allows them to be proactive in their relationships. Imagine that you and a friend are driving home after a weekend of camping. You run out of gas on a lonely road. Your friend immediately begins to panic, fearing that she is in danger. You remain calm, remembering that this happened to you once before and that a neighbor came to your aid. Your confidence can "rub off" on your friend, helping her to realize that the situation will probably end positively.

Conclusion

People who are emotionally healthy are mindful of the emotions they experience. They realize that their emotions affect their quality of life and their relationships. They learn to express their emotions in constructive ways that help them accomplish goals and maintain relationships. Finally, they remember that emotions are a call to action. They find ways to use the energy of emotions to enhance their lives.

Discussion Questions

1. How are emotions related to energy?
2. Name an emotion you experienced lately. What caused it? How are you able to recognize that emotion?

3. Consider an emotion. List as many synonyms for that emotion as possible.
4. Consider techniques you could employ to utilize emotions.

References

American Academy of Family Physicians. (2002). *Mental health: Keeping your emotional health.* Retrieved January 19, 2006, from http://www.familydoctor.org

Barnhart, R. K. (ed.). (1988). *The Barnhart dictionary of etymology.* Bronx, NY: H.W. Wilson.

Breuss, C. E., & Richardson, G. E. (1994). *Healthy decisions.* Madison, WI: Brown & Benchmark.

Chantrell, C. (ed.). (2002). *The Oxford dictionary of word histories.* Oxford: Oxford University Press.

Donatelle, R. J. (2006). *Access to health* (9th ed.). San Francisco: Pearson Benjamin Cummings.

Edlin, G., & Golanty, E. (2007). *Health and wellness* (9th ed.). Sudbury, MA: Jones and Bartlett.

Ekman, P. (2003). *Emotions revealed: Recognizing faces and feelings to improve communication and emotional life.* New York: Times.

Feinstein, J. (2006). *Last dance: Behind the scenes at the final four.* New York: Little, Brown.

Floyd, P. A., Mimms, S. E, & Yelding, C. (2003). *Personal health: Perspectives and lifestyles* (3rd ed.). Belmont, CA: Thomson Wadsworth.

Funk & Wagnalls New International Dictionary of the English Language. (1989). New York: J. G. Ferguson.

Goleman, D. (1995). *Emotional intelligence: Why it can matter more than IQ.* New York: Bantam.

Goleman, D. (1998). *Working with emotional intelligence.* New York: Bantam.

Hunter, E. M. (2004). *Little book of big emotions: How five feelings affect everything you do (and don't do).* Center City, MN: Hazelden.

Insel, P. M. & Roth, W. T. (2004). *Core concepts in health* (9th ed.). Boston: McGraw-Hill.

Knapp, C. (1996). *Drinking: A love story.* New York: Dial Press.

Myers, D. G. (2001). *Exploring psychology* (6th ed.). New York: Worth.

Payne, W. A., & Hahn, D. B. (2002). *Understanding your health* (7th ed.). Boston: McGraw-Hill.

Salovey, P., & Mayer, J. D. (1990). Emotional intelligence. *Imagination, Cognition and Personality, 9*(3), 185–211.

Scandurra, A. J. (1999). Everyday spirituality: A core unit in health education and lifetime wellness. *Journal of Health Education, 30*(2), 104–109.

Seaward, B. L. (2001). *Health of the human spirit: Spiritual dimensions for personal health.* Boston: Allyn & Bacon.

Steiner, C. (1997). *Achieving emotional literacy: A personal program to increase your emotional intelligence.* New York: Avon.

Thomas, D. Q., & Kotecki, J. E. (2007). *Physical activity and health* (2nd ed.). Sudbury, MA: Jones and Bartlett.

Turner, L. W., Sizer, F. S., Whitney, E. N., & Wilks, B. B. (1992). *Life choices: Health concepts and strategies.* St. Paul, MN: West.

CHAPTER 5 ▶

Intellectual Health

Nothing in life is to be feared. It is only to be understood.

—Marie Curie, 1944

Whenever we think, we think for a purpose within a point of view based on assumptions leading to implications and consequences. We use ideas and theories to interpret data, facts, and experiences in order to answer questions, solve problems, and resolve issues.

— Richard Paul & Linda Elder, 2001

Introduction

What is the intellect? For many years the terms *intellect* and *intelligence* have been used interchangeably to refer to the higher thinking centers of the brain. More recently "intelligence" has been used to mean a variety of things. Harvard psychologist Howard Gardner (1999), for example, has popularized the idea of "multiple intelligences." He believes that different people learn best in different ways. Some examples of these intelligences are linguistic, logical-mathematical, musical, and bodily-kinesthetic. Psychologist Daniel Goleman (1995) has written a book titled *Emotional Intelligence* focusing on our feelings and how we can use them to help identify appropriate behaviors in certain situations. Thus, the concept of intelligence has broadened considerably. We can no longer limit its use to intellectual capacities.

The word *intellect* can be traced back to two Latin words (Barnhart, 1988; Chantrell, 2002). *Intellectus* refers to "understanding or discernment," and was derived from the verb *intellegere* meaning "to choose from." The implication of the verb form is that the intellect is important in decision making. We can use

The brain is the master organ for
intellectual health.

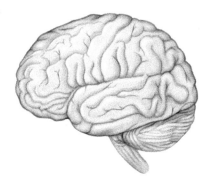

our intellect to weigh the pros and cons in a particular situation and choose the
best course of action. Imagine that you are thinking about joining a health club.
You might make lists of the disadvantages and benefits. The cost of member-
ship might be a problem. However, additional motivation to work out might be
a positive.

This famous statue in Paris
reflects the importance we place
on intellectual health.

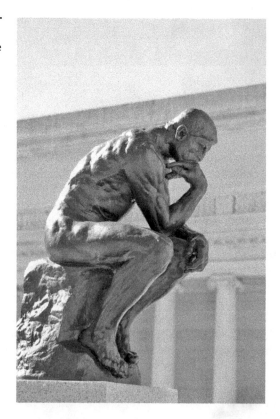

"Intelligence" or IQ tests have focused on "verbal memory, verbal reasoning, numerical reasoning, appreciation of logical sequences, and ability to state how one would solve problems of daily living" (Gardner, 1999). They are really attempts to measure intellectual capabilities.

Psychologist and philosopher Mortimer Adler (1990) argues that although intellectual processes are dependent on the brain, these processes are immaterial in nature. Thus the intellect is an "immaterial component of human nature" (p. xi). He suggests that intellect is the "highest power" humans possess (p. 3). Furthermore, he contends that other animals have minds, but that they do not have intellectual powers. These uniquely human powers include the "ability to conceive or understand, the ability to make judgments, and the ability to reason or make inferences" (p. 8).

You may wonder why your ability to think and understand is a component of your health. Two simple arguments can be made for the inclusion of the intellectual dimension in a model of health. First, remember that *health* deals with optimal functioning of the whole person. Clearly our ability to learn, think, and make decisions is a significant aspect of human functioning. Second, we are bombarded every day with new health research. Sometimes these studies contradict one another. We need to have the ability to evaluate that information critically in order to adopt healthful behaviors.

Definitions and Descriptions of Intellectual Health

Dianne Hales is a well-respected health author who has written several popular college health textbooks. According to Hales (2009), intellectual health "refers to your ability to think and learn from life experiences, your openness to new ideas, and your capacity to question and evaluate information" (p. 7). She also mentions that critical thinking skills are necessary throughout your life. Edlin and Golanty (2007) also emphasize open-mindedness, suggesting that the intellectually healthy person has "a mind open to new ideas and concepts" (p. 11).

Donatelle (2005) of Oregon State University describes intellectual health as the "ability to think clearly, reason objectively, analyze critically, and use brain power effectively to meet life's challenges" (p. 4). Alters and Schiff (2009) agree when they write that "intellectual health is the ability to use problem-solving and other higher-order thinking skills to deal effectively with life's challenges" (p. 3).

Dr. Elaine de Beauport is a teacher and researcher, as well as founder of the Mead School for Human Development, which emphasizes development of the whole child. Dr. de Beauport's (1996) definition of "rational intelligence" is "to reason, explain, and connect thoughts sequentially and logically" (p. 345). She believes that this is only one aspect of intellectual health—there are other types of thinking that utilize the neocortex.

Intellectual health has also been defined as "the ability to process and act on information, clarify values and beliefs, and exercise decision-making capacity"

Asking questions
improves knowledge
and intellectual health.

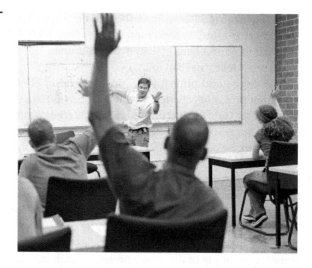

(Payne & Hahn, 2002, p. 18). Ball State University professors Payne and Hahn continue by suggesting that the ability to use information and to grasp new ideas is particularly important for students to succeed.

Psychologist David Myers (2005) of Hope College uses the term *intelligence* in the way we have used *intellect*. His definition is "the mental abilities needed to select, adapt to, and shape environments. It involves the abilities to profit from experience, solve problems, reason, and successfully meet challenges and achieve goals" (p. 315).

These experts from a variety of disciplines have identified many variables. However, you can see some overlapping ideas. Reasoning, problem solving, making connections, and clear thinking are present in more than one description.

Models of Intellectual Health

Although virtually all models of health include an intellectual dimension, little attention has been given to this dimension in the health education literature. The tendency in textbooks is to briefly define intellectual health in the introductory chapter and then ignore it. Therefore, the models presented here originate in other disciplines. Education and psychology have focused much attention on learning and the intellect. We will examine ideas from these disciplines and apply them to optimal thinking, that is, intellectual health.

Cognitive Development Model

Jean Piaget was one of the most influential psychologists of the twentieth century (Myers, 2005). He assumed that we are continually trying to understand the

Sensorimotor ——► Preoperational ——► Concrete operations ——► Formal operations

Cognitive Stages of Development.

world and people around us and that we are "actively involved in learning and interpreting events" (Ormrod, 1995, p. 173). During the 1920s Piaget identified stages of cognitive development. Cognition refers to "all the mental activities associated with thinking, knowing, remembering, and communicating" (Myers, 2005, p. 128). He theorized that our capacities for thinking, learning, and understanding mature as we grow and develop. Although modern psychologists believe the development is more gradual and perhaps earlier than Piaget proposed, his stages are valid for most individuals.

SENSORIMOTOR STAGE

Understanding of the environment is limited to what is experienced through the senses and motor interactions with objects. Children can only think about what is literally in front of them until they are about 2 years old. The phrase "out of sight, out of mind" describes this level of thinking. If you are playing with an infant and put the teddy bear behind your back, the infant will immediately forget about it. They lack *object permanence*. When the child matures, she will look for the teddy bear behind your back.

PREOPERATIONAL STAGE

This stage lasts from age 2 until age 6 or 7. The crucial aspects of this stage are appearance of language and the ability to think about things in their absence. However, some mental operations are illogical by adult standards. For example, a classic experiment involves the concept of *conservation*. The child is presented with a tall glass of liquid and then watches while the liquid is poured into a short, squat glass. Children in the preoperational stage will report that the tall glass holds more liquid.

STAGE OF CONCRETE OPERATIONS

This stage lasts until age 11 or 12. By now children understand ideas such as conservation of a liquid. However, children in this stage can use logic only with concrete, observable objects and events. They understand that a 5-pound dumbbell weighs the same as five 1-pound dumbbells.

STAGE OF FORMAL OPERATIONS

This stage rarely appears before age 11 and develops for several years. It includes the ability to reason with abstract, hypothetical, and contrary-to-fact information.

During this stage children are able to understand and test hypotheses. They understand *if-then* relationships.

Thinking abilities develop as humans mature. Infants can perceive only what they see, hear, or feel. Older children and adults can reason using images or even information that doesn't make sense.

Dimensions of Thinking Model

The Association for Supervision and Curriculum Development (ASCD) sponsored an attempt to help educators understand and teach thinking. The result was a book titled *Dimensions of Thinking* (Marzano et al., 1988). The authors reviewed the literature and developed a framework for understanding how people think. The goal was to help the schools teach students to think. The five dimensions of thinking are: (1) metacognition, (2) critical and creative thinking, (3) thinking processes, (4) core thinking skills, and (5) the relationship of content-area knowledge to thinking.

METACOGNITION

The first dimension of thinking refers to our "awareness and control of our own thinking" (Marzano et al, 1988, p. 4). Your beliefs about yourself and your values will influence the motivation and effort given to any task. Metacognition includes a commitment to the task, your attitude about the importance or value of the task, and "executive control," which includes evaluation, planning, and regulation.

CRITICAL AND CREATIVE THINKING

Most thinking involves one or both of these components. They are complementary and overlapping rather than discrete ways of thinking. Ennis describes critical thinking as "reasonable, reflective thinking that is focused on deciding what to believe or do" (Marzano et al., 1988, p. 18). Critical thinkers ask questions, analyze arguments, judge the credibility of sources, and make decisions based on information and their evaluation of that information. Imagine that you want to start a diet. Before you choose one, you ask about the benefits and possible dangers, you examine the credentials of the authors, and then you choose one that you expect will be safe and effective.

Halpern describes creative thinking as "the ability to form new combinations of ideas to fulfill a need" (Marzano et al., 1988, p. 23). Creative thinking requires output. Without results there is no evidence of creative thinking. Creative thinkers are willing to take risks and possess the ability to evaluate themselves. They are willing to push the limits of their knowledge and application, and they trust their own abilities in this quest. Creative thinking may be enhanced by letting ideas flow when not focused on the problem at hand. Some people, for example, have their best ideas while exercising. The activity requires involvement of the body and the mind is left to wander. Cardiokickboxing is a result of creative thinking. The developers took a risk by combining martial arts with aerobic movements, and a new exercise craze was born.

THINKING PROCESSES

Marzano et al. (1988) identify two thinking processes. The first is knowledge acquisition. You can gain knowledge through formation of concepts and principles and via comprehension. Comprehension involves interpreting information and relating it to what you already know. The second process is knowledge production and application. Scientific research is one example of knowledge production, and problem solving applies that knowledge. When you study a new discipline you must learn the vocabulary. If you are learning about aerobic exercise, you must learn to classify different activities as aerobic based on common characteristics. Then you can apply this knowledge as you devise your personal exercise program.

CORE THINKING SKILLS

These skills are necessary for the other dimensions of thinking. They might be considered micro-processes or prerequisites to the more complex thinking processes described previously. Core thinking skills are a means to achieve the goals of the other dimensions of thinking. Marzano et al. (1988) identify several core thinking skills, including information gathering, organizing, remembering, analyzing, integrating, and evaluating. You *gather* information through observation; you *organize* and *remember* by encoding, classifying, and ordering. *Analysis* involves identifying attributes, relationships, main ideas, and errors. *Integration* requires you to summarize. Finally, *evaluating* requires criteria to use as standards. You can't evaluate your sexual behavior without some criteria for healthful behavior.

RELATIONSHIP OF CONTENT-AREA KNOWLEDGE TO THINKING

Thinking does not occur in a vacuum. You cannot just think critically. This dimension assumes you have some knowledge of the material you are thinking about. It provides context for the other four dimensions of thinking.

A fundamental aspect of these dimensions is that they may occur simultaneously. While deciding whether to exercise (metacognition), you might be considering what type of exercise you prefer (critical/creative thinking), while simultaneously thinking about whether you have enough time to finish your workout (thinking processes), and whether you really want to change clothes and shower (core thinking skills).

Intellectual activity
occurs in the brain.

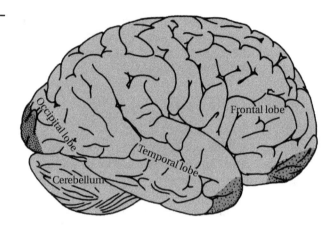

Faces of Mind Model

Elaine de Beauport is an educator and researcher. Her book *The Three Faces of Mind* (de Beauport, 1996) is based on research indicating that there are three levels of the neocortex (the higher brain centers). Intellectual activity occurs in the neocortex. It is the "brain system that distinguishes us as human beings from all other forms of life. It permits us to make distinctions and reflect on our thoughts, feelings, and actions as human beings" (p. 5). Function of the neocortex can be divided into four realms or ways of knowing: rational, associative, spatial, and intuitive. These four intelligences of the neocortex form de Beauport's model of intellectual health.

RATIONAL INTELLIGENCE

Sequential, precise, and logical connections result from rational thinking. Rational thought seeks reasons for what we experience, links between cause and effect, and critical differences. Rational thinkers often ask the classic questions who, what, when, where, how, and why. This type of thought is highly valued in Western cultures. The scientific method is the application of rational intelligence. Scientists search for critical differences between variables to establish cause–effect relationships. This leads to understanding and more questions to study. The process is repeated and the body of knowledge grows. Rational thinking assumes that one or more causes exist for every situation.

Although de Beauport (1996) values rational intelligence, she believes that too often we stop halfway through the process. She suggests that we tend to stop thinking about a problem once we understand its cause. Instead we should complete the process by finding solutions to the problem. Comprehension is not enough. We need to invent or create. Understanding occurs when we have carefully looked at all the parts of the problem. However, the process is not complete until we act to improve the situation. There must be both a discovery phase and a solution phase. If you feel tired all the time, you can examine the situation and determine the causes of your tiredness. But the process is not complete until you invent and try new ways to increase energy levels during the day.

ASSOCIATIVE INTELLIGENCE

Rational intelligence involves sequential thinking; however, sometimes we achieve an understanding without worrying about sequences. This may occur through juxtaposition, associations, and relationships. Thinking relationally is not a substitute for rational thinking. It is an alternative way of thinking. The associations are related to people, places, ideas, objects, colors, and concepts. Without concern for cause and effect, the associative thinker is free to discover without need for conclusions or judgments. Often the connections seem random. Brainstorming is a popular example of associative thinking. For example, a teacher might ask a class, "What are stressors in your life?" Students respond with answers that are not surprising—money, roommates, tests, and so on. But one student replies "peanuts." It turns out she is allergic to peanuts. This response may turn the discussion in an entirely new direction. Brainstorming is clearly not sequential. Yet that type of thinking can be very useful in helping people change paradigms and yielding entirely new ways of thinking about or studying a topic.

Associative thinking is useful in many situations. For example, a scientist may be thinking about a problem and "gets a glimpse" of some reality; she "sees" a new relationship. She then sets up her hypothesis and proceeds to test it using rational processes. Building relationships also depends on associative intelligence. You cannot think sequentially about people. As you come in contact with someone, you are bombarded by a variety of stimuli—the person's words, appearance, mood, clothing, and posture may all affect you. de Beauport (1996) suggests that associative intelligence allows us to respond to that which interests us. This process allows connections to develop between people. Associative intelligence may also be the type of thinking that allows an addict to overcome denial. The typical thinking of an addict is "I have so many problems, I deserve a drink." The alcoholic who ends up in recovery at some point turns those associations around (juxtaposition) and says, "I drink too much and that causes many of my problems." Once that reversal of thinking occurs, the addict is ready to say, "My life is unbearable. I need help."

SPATIAL INTELLIGENCE

Imagination uses deeper portions of the neocortex. You can visualize instructions, people, and events in the future. Using your brain to create images helps you to develop and remember connections between events and people. We use external input from the senses, as well as internal input from emotions. Spatial intelligence builds connections using this information. The best listeners are patient enough to wait and understand the message someone is sending. These listeners can also interpret visual cues about meaning. They study facial expressions and posture. They can then connect inner meanings to the sounds they heard.

INTUITIVE INTELLIGENCE

Intuition is "knowing from within, knowing without recourse to logic or reason" (de Beauport, 1996, p. 62). de Beauport suggests that intuition is what we have "named spirituality, something far beyond what we are used to calling 'intelligence'" (p. 61). de Beauport believes that we need to embrace intuition in our daily lives. We need to trust our gut feelings. Don't be afraid of your best hunch, even if you cannot explain it.

You may have heard the phrase the "art and science of medicine." The "science" is, of course, rational intelligence; however, the "art" refers to intuition. Sometimes the doctor "just knows" what the illness might be or how to treat it. This may occur without having treated the condition before. They "face the unknown" and a solution appears to them. This is especially important for pediatricians and veterinarians whose patients have limited ability to communicate with them.

These models demonstrate that thinking occurs in different ways such as rational and associative. It also has different goals such as problem solving and knowing for the sake of knowing.

Characteristics of Intellectually Healthy People

Donatelle (2005) provides a checklist for intellectual health. She suggests that intellectually healthy people consider options and consequences, learn from mistakes, avoid risks, are informed consumers, have hobbies that provide personal growth, manage time effectively, and examine evidence regarding perceptions and opinions.

Floyd et al. (2008) suggest several indicators of intellectual health. These attributes are alertness, creativity, logic, curiosity, open-mindedness, and a keen memory.

Insel and Roth (2004) believe that intellectual wellness is characterized by open-mindedness, the ability to question and think critically, the desire to learn new skills, a sense of humor, creativity, and curiosity.

Alters and Schiff (2009) write that intellectually healthy people "analyze situations, determine alternative courses of action, and make decisions" and that they can "judge the effectiveness of their choices and learn from their experiences" (p. 3).

Paul and Elder (2001) suggest that effective thinkers achieve "activated knowledge." This means that they recognize and use true knowledge. Activated thinking then results in more questions as we understand the knowledge we have. Active thinkers seek principles that underlie whatever topic they are learning about; they

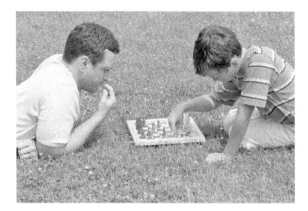

Hobbies can exercise the brain.

search for underlying laws and theories. Thus, their knowledge is contextual. It is not random bits or memorized facts that are disconnected from life. The authors also assert that active thinkers ask questions. They are driven more by questions than answers. Bernd Heinrich (2001) wrote a book about his personal training program for a 62-mile ultramarathon race. Heinrich is a biologist at the University of Vermont. He used his knowledge of "ultramarathoning" animals such as migratory birds to inform his own training for the race. Each bit of information was contextual. He evaluated the context of the animals to see how their activities and physiology were similar to his. Then he developed a training program that incorporated appropriate knowledge from those animals. So, his own context became a second barometer to evaluate, ask questions, and apply knowledge. Paul and Elder contend that "to question is to learn well."

Ennis (Marzano et al., 1988) lists the following characteristics as he focuses on critical thinking: seeks reasons; is well-informed; uses credible sources for decision making; is open-minded; looks for alternatives; and is sensitive to others' feelings, knowledge, and sophistication.

A New Model of Intellectual Health

Identifying themes is difficult when the origins of the information are diverse and the vocabulary varies. However, a three-component sequential model does emerge after identifying the recurring themes in the definitions and models. The first component is *knowledge acquisition*. However, acquisition is not enough. Knowledge must be understood to be useful. Therefore, *comprehension* is the second component. Intellectual health requires understanding and context, not just the accumulation of discrete facts. Finally, for a person to be intellectually healthy, they must *apply* the knowledge. Although we may hear the phrase "knowledge for its own sake," even that value has purpose. It is to "exercise" the

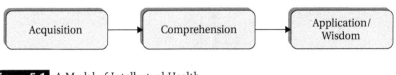

Figure 5.1 A Model of Intellectual Health

intellect and perhaps to provide a foundation and context for future intellectual activity. Wisdom is the highest level of application. **Figure 5.1** illustrates this developmental model.

Acquisition of Knowledge

Learning requires motivation. We can be motivated either internally or externally. Internal motivation involves a love of learning or curiosity. Sometimes we simply wonder about things. We don't expect any practical benefit from the knowledge gained. One summer the author hired a professional to remove bats from his home. A friend happened to be visiting one day when the "bat man" arrived to check his traps. The friend peppered him with questions for almost 30 minutes. He wanted to know where they winter, how they reproduce, how long they live, and so on. The friend is curious about the world. Curiosity may be specific (e.g., only about bats) or global, a "wide-eyed approach to everything" (Seligman, 2002, p. 141).

External motivation is needs-based. Necessity drives external motivation. You may be preparing for the comprehensive exam in your major. You need to pass in order to graduate. Or, you may take a part-time job that requires specific training and knowledge. These are examples of external motivation. It is practical. There is something to be gained by knowing.

We can acquire knowledge in a variety of ways. Sometimes we memorize facts. To do this we may repeat them over and over, or we may use flashcards. The goal is to "force" knowledge into our heads. Another type of acquisition is concept formation. Forming concepts involves organizing information so we can discriminate between particular objects or ideas. For example, by the end of a fitness class you should be able to identify different strength training activities by their common characteristics. At the end of a communicable disease unit, you should be able to recognize different types of pathogens. A crucial component of concept formation is vocabulary. We use words to symbolize concepts. Therefore, knowledge of vocabulary is the foundation of concept formation. At the highest level of concept formation you should be able to "identify examples of the concept, name the concept and its distinguishing attributes, give a societally accepted definition of the concept, and indicate how examples of the concept differ from nonexamples" (Marzano et al., 1988, p. 36).

Another type of knowledge acquisition is principle formation. Principle formation occurs when you organize concepts into relationships. This process helps organize information into disciplines. Several types of principles exist. *Cause-and-effect* principles have "if-then" meanings; "HIV causes AIDS" is one example. *Correlational* principles identify relationships in which a change in one state is predictably related to a change in a second variable; for example, "Big people tend to be stronger." No cause–effect relationship has been established. *Axiomatic* principles are universally accepted truths. "Exercise is good for your health" illustrates an axiom.

Acquisition of knowledge is the first step toward intellectual health. Acquisition provides the foundation for the other components of intellectual health.

Comprehension of Knowledge

Knowing is necessary, but not sufficient for intellectual health. Sometimes we know facts, but are unable to put them in context. You may remember a time when you just memorized information for an exam, but you didn't really understand it. Comprehension requires you to know more than the fact that average blood pressure is 120/80 mm Hg. You also need to understand what systolic blood pressure is and how it affects your health. If you had to teach it to someone else, you could explain the significance of blood pressure. Comprehension focuses on understanding. You can recite the information and also explain it. You can see how it fits into a greater whole. When you comprehend information, it has meaning for you. When you comprehend you integrate new information with what you already know. For example, you may learn about the distinction between exercise and physical activity. If exercise has always been associated with jogging, pain, and a large time commitment, new information about the benefits of physical activity can give it new meaning. You may realize that you don't have to be "athletic" or that you don't even have to sweat to improve your physical health. Thus, comprehension requires interpretation.

Many strategies have been proposed to enhance comprehension. Reciprocal teaching, for example, requires you to teach your classmates by summarizing important data, asking questions about the information, and clarifying misunderstandings.

Application of Knowledge

As de Beauport (1996) suggests, gaining knowledge and attaching meaning to it are valuable, but the process is still not complete. You must also use the knowledge. Problem solving is a crucial element of application. Humans must solve problems in order to survive. Problem solving occurs on a global level as scientists search for new energy sources, but it also occurs in more mundane ways as you learn your way around a new university campus or try to figure out what went wrong on last night's date. Some problem-solving strategies are sequential in nature. The IDEAL process developed by Bransford and Stein (Marzano et al.,

1988) is an example. IDEAL stands for Identify the problem, Define the problem, Explore strategies for solving the problem, Act on the ideas, Look for effects. Other strategies provide unordered suggestions like: (1) get the big picture, (2) withhold judgment, (3) state the question in different forms, (4) try working backwards, (5) use analogies and metaphors (Marzano et al.).

A closely related application of knowledge is decision making. Decision making requires you to choose between two or more options or to invent an alternative that is better according to some criteria. Identifying the criteria also requires a decision. Health educators Meeks and Heit (1992) have proposed the following "Responsible Decision Making Model" for school-age children:

1. Clearly describe the situation.
2. Make a list of possible actions that could be taken.
3. Share your list of possible actions with a responsible adult.
4. Carefully evaluate each possible action using six criteria.
   a. Will this decision result in an action that promotes my health and the health of others?
   b. Will this decision result in an action that protects my safety and the safety of others?
   c. Will this decision result in an action that protects the laws of the community?
   d. Will this decision result in an action that shows respect for myself and others?
   e. Will this decision result in an action that follows guidelines set by responsible adults such as parents?
   f. Will this decision result in an action that demonstrates that I have good character and moral values?
5. Decide which action is responsible and most appropriate.
6. Act in a responsible way and evaluate the results.

You can see that this is a very rational, linear approach to decision making and that the authors had to engage in their own decision making as they identified the six criteria for responsible decisions. And notice that step six requires application.

A third way to apply knowledge is composition. This may sound like writing, and in education it often is. Composition is broader than that, however. It is the process of "conceiving and developing a product" (Marzano et al., 1988). It may mean developing an aerobic dance routine, writing and performing a play about healthy relationships, or creating a PowerPoint presentation about sexually transmitted infections. Composition often requires activity. It has been said that we learn best by doing.

Flower and Hayes (Marzano et al., 1988, p. 57) have developed a theory of composition for writing; however, it may be adapted to the process of composition in general. They believe that composition incorporates three operations: (1) planning, (2) translating, and (3) reviewing. During planning the composer organizes information, sets goals, and generates ideas. Translation puts ideas into understandable language (or other symbols). In the case of developing an aerobic dance workout, the ideas are translated into specific movements that will accomplish the goals set out. Reviewing, of course, involves evaluating and revising. The composer will actually perform the aerobics routine to see if it achieves its goals: Is the routine aerobic? Is the duration sufficient? Does the exerciser reach the target heart rate? Do the moves flow smoothly from one into the next? Based on this evaluation, the composer will revise the routine. Sometimes the review is less formal. Perhaps the composer will develop a feeling that it "just isn't working." Perhaps different songs will then be considered to see if they better fit the patterns in or the pace of the routine.

We may have "aha" moments when pieces of information fit together. Sometimes these "aha" moments occur while learning skills, too. For example, Joe enrolled in a 5-day sailing class. For the first 4 days he was lost. He knew the facts, the information about sailing, but couldn't put it into practice. He couldn't figure out where the wind was coming from. When he tried to come about (turn), he lost control of the boat. But on the last day (just in time for the practical test), he got it. He sailed the course like a pro—no mistakes.

Wisdom is the highest level of application and has many definitions. The *New International Dictionary of the English Language* (Funk & Wagnalls, 1987) provides a sample:

> 1. the power of true and right discernment: conformity to the course of action dictated by such discernment. 2. good practical judgment; common sense. 3. a high degree of knowledge; learning. (p. 1445)

The dictionary (Funk & Wagnalls, 1987) then lists many synonyms including enlightenment, erudition, foresight, insight, judgment, judiciousness, sagacity, and understanding. Snodgrass (2004) states that the wise person is able to "read a situation and make the appropriate decisions for right living" (p. 38). The wise person is able to discern and make sound judgments and recommendations. You can count on the wise to give good advice in difficult situations. An assumption is that wisdom involves moral decisions, judgments that are "good."

Kitchner and Brenner (1990) suggest that wisdom has four components: (1) presence of difficult or "thorny" problems, (2) appropriate knowledge characterized by both breadth and depth, (3) recognition that knowledge is uncertain and that no one knows the whole truth, and (4) willingness and ability to devise "sound, executable judgments in the face of this uncertainty" (p. 213). Wise people are sought out because they have the background knowledge related to the problem at hand and they are able and willing to use that knowledge to make recommendations about behavior.

Conclusion

Intellectual health contributes to the well-being of the whole person. It requires us to think and learn. We think and learn about life, about health, about relationships, and about our purpose in life. Without analyzing, making connections, and solving problems, we would not reach our full potential as humans.

Discussion Questions

1. What do you think about when you are free to let your mind wander?
2. List techniques you use to acquire knowledge.
3. Does comprehension automatically occur when you acquire knowledge? Explain.
4. List examples of how people have applied their knowledge to make life better for themselves or others.

References

Adler, M. (1990). *Intellect: Mind over matter*. New York: Macmillan.

Alters, S., & Schiff, W. (2009). *Essential concepts for healthy living* (5th ed.). Sudbury, MA: Jones and Bartlett.

Barnhart, R. K. (ed.). (1988). *The Barnhart dictionary of etymology*. New York: H.W. Wilson.

Chantrell, C. (ed.). (2002). *The Oxford dictionary of word histories*. Oxford, England: Oxford University Press.

de Beauport, E. (1996). *The three faces of mind: Developing your mental, emotional, and behavioral intelligences*. Wheaton, IL: Quest.

Donatelle, R. J. (2005). *Health: The basics* (6th ed.). San Francisco: Pearson Benjamin Cummings.

Edlin, G., & Golanty, E. (2007). *Health and wellness* (9th ed.). Sudbury, MA: Jones and Bartlett.

Floyd, P. A., Mimms, S. E., & Yelding, C. (2008). *Personal health: Perspectives and lifestyles* (4th ed.). Belmont, CA: Thomson Wadsworth.

Funk & Wagnalls New International Dictionary of the English Language. (1987). Chicago: J. G. Ferguson.

Gardner, H. (1999). *Intelligence reframed: Multiple intelligences for the 21st century*. New York: Basic.

Goleman, D. (1995). *Emotional intelligence: Why it can matter more than IQ*. New York: Bantam.

Hales, D. (2009). *An invitation to health*. Belmont, CA: Wadsworth Cengage Learning.

Heinrich, B. (2001). *Racing the antelope: What animals can teach us about racing and life*. New York: Cliff Street.

Insel, P. M., & Roth, W. T. (2004). *Core concepts in health* (9th ed.). Boston: McGraw-Hill.

Kitchner, K. S., & Brenner, H. G. (1990). Wisdom and reflective judgment: Knowing in the face of uncertainty. In R. J. Sternberg (Ed.), *Wisdom: Its nature, origins, and development* (pp. 212–229). Cambridge: Cambridge University Press.

Marzano, R. J., Brandt, R. S., Hughes, C. S., Jones, B. F., Presseisen, B. Z., Rankin, S. C., et al. (1988). *Dimensions of thinking: A framework for curriculum and instruction.* Alexandria, VA: Association for Supervision and Curriculum Development.

Meeks, L., & Heit, P. (1992). *Comprehensive school health education.* Blacklick, OH: Meeks-Heit.

Myers, D. G. (2005) *Exploring psychology* (6th ed.). New York: Worth.

Ormrod, J. E. (1995). *Human learning* (2nd ed.). Englewood Cliffs, NJ: Merrill.

Paul, R., & Elder, L. (2001). *A miniature guide for students on how to study and learn a discipline using critical thinking concepts and tools.* Dillon Beach, CA: Foundation for Critical Thinking.

Payne, W. A., & Hahn, D. B. (2002). *Understanding your health* (7th ed.). Boston: McGraw-Hill.

Seligman, M. E. P. (2002). *Authentic happiness: Using the new positive psychology to realize your potential for lasting fulfillment.* New York: Free Press.

Snodgrass, K. (2004). *Between two truths: Living with Biblical tensions.* Eugene, OR: Wipf & Stock.

CHAPTER 6 ▶

Spiritual Health

The spiritual dimension is your core, your center, your commitment to your value system.

—Stephen Covey, 1989

Introduction

Students have school spirit. A horse with lots of energy is spirited. Debates are sometimes referred to as spirited discussions. These applications of the word *spirit* don't really get to the heart of its meaning, however. The word *spirit* is derived from the Latin words *spiritus* meaning "breath, courage, vigor, or soul" and *spirare* to breathe (Barnhart, 1988; Chantrell, 2002). Humans must breathe to survive. The human spirit refers to the life-giving aspect or core of an individual. Spiritual health is essential to well-being. Some models of health place the spiritual dimension at the center or over and above the other dimensions (Banks, 1980; Russell, 1987), indicating the crucial role that spiritual health plays. Russell views the spiritual dimension as overarching, the component of health that provides context for all other dimensions.

Bensley (1991) of Central Michigan University reviewed definitions of spiritual health. He identified six different perspectives on spiritual health: (1) fulfillment in life, (2) values and beliefs, (3) wholeness, (4) a component of health, (5) God or a higher power, and (6) the human/spiritual interaction. These perspectives are not mutually exclusive. Some are personal, some are social, and some are related to characteristics that transcend humanity. Bensley asserts that the lack of consensus regarding a definition of spiritual health makes research into the topic difficult. A sample of these definitions is presented later in this chapter. You will see that different concepts of spiritual health still exist.

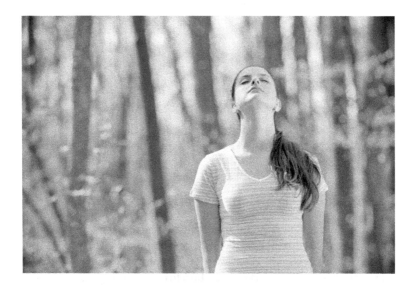

Prayer and meditation can improve spiritual health.

One area of confusion is the relationship between spiritual health (or spirituality) and religion. Some people equate the two; however, distinctions can be made. Religion tends to be an institution. It is organized and incorporates specific rituals and behaviors. Seaward (2001) describes religion as a "commitment to a specific observance of your faith" (p. 78). Most often religion seeks a relationship with God or a higher being. Religion is communal in nature; people gather to practice their religion. Spirituality is less organized and more free-flowing with fewer rules and expectations. Spirituality seeks answers to questions such as "Who am I?" and "Why am I here?" It may be communal or personal.

A person may attend worship services regularly but not really accept or live by the beliefs of that religion. That is, he or she may be religious, but not very spiritual. For example, a friend described attending church every Sunday as a child, but never realizing that church services and faith were related to what he did during the week. On the other hand, some people never attend formal worship services or associate themselves with organized religion. Yet they might believe in God, feel fulfilled in their lives, have a strong sense of purpose, or find fulfillment in helping others or spending time in nature.

Seaward (2001) believes that religion is intended and able to promote spiritual growth. The two are compatible, but not identical. He envisions two overlapping circles. Thus a person may be (1) religious but not spiritual, (2) spiritual but not religious, or (3) spiritual and religious (see **Figure 6.1**).

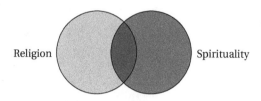

Figure 6.1 The Relationship Between Religion and Spirituality

Definitions and Descriptions of Spiritual Health

Bloomfield and Kory (1978) contend that "spiritual health generates a sense of personal fulfillment, a sense of peace with yourself and the world" (p. 244).

Health author Dianne Hales (2009) writes that "spiritually healthy individuals identify their own basic purpose in life; learn how to experience love, joy, peace, and fulfillment; and help themselves and others achieve their full potential" (p. 6).

"Spiritual wellness combines a person's ethics, values, and morals. This component is what gives life meaning and purpose. It is based on faith, hope, love, optimism, and forgiveness," according to Floyd, Mimms, and Yelding (2008, p. 2) of Alabama State University. Young (1984) incorporates similar ideas, describing spiritual health as "an ongoing process of growth in three areas—faith, hope, and love" (p. 279).

Breuss and Richardson (1994, p. 6) are both university health educators and professors. They don't define spiritual health, but they envision it as a continuum with peak experiences at one end and guilt or lack of purpose at the other. Peak experiences indicate optimal spiritual health, and guilt or lack of purpose demonstrates poor spiritual health.

Insel and Roth (2004) of Stanford University write that spiritually healthy people "possess a set of guiding beliefs, principles, or values that give meaning and purpose to your life" (p. 2).

Byer and Shainberg (1995) are from Mt. San Antonio College. They propose three components of spiritual health: "seeing yourself as part of a 'larger scheme of things,' having a sense of purpose on earth, and feeling concern for the well-being of other people" (p. 11). They later state that spirituality unifies the various aspects of our lives to make a "meaningful whole," brings focus and meaning, and allows connections to form between people. Donatelle (2005), a professor at Oregon Stage University, also recognizes the unifying aspect of spiritual health, describing this component as "a belief in a unifying force that gives meaning to life and transcends the purely physical or personal dimensions of existence" (p. 34).

Scandurra (1999) is a health educator at DePaul University who has developed a spiritual health unit for health education classes. She believes that spiritual

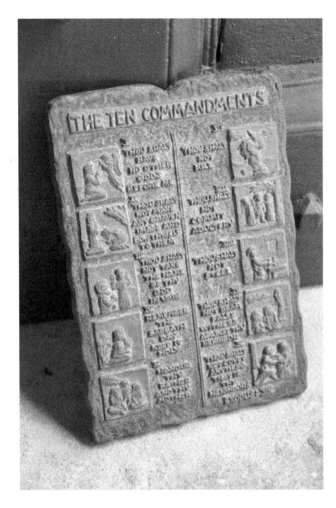

Religious belief
and practice can
enhance spiritual
health.

health includes "connectedness to oneself, others, nature, and to a larger meaning or purpose" (p. 104). Personal characteristics that contribute to the development of spiritual health are creativity, play, love, forgiveness, compassion, trust, reverence, wisdom, and faith.

Hawks (1994), a health educator at Utah State University, defines spiritual health as "a high level of faith, hope, and commitment in relation to a well-defined worldview or belief system that provides a sense of meaning and purpose to existence in general, and that offers an ethical path to personal fulfillment which includes connectedness with self, others, and a higher power or larger reality" (p. 4).

Alters and Schiff (2009) define spiritual health as "the belief that one is a part of a larger scheme of life and that one's life has purpose" (p. 3). They suggest that for

Box 6.1	Common Elements of Spiritual Health
Values	Forgiveness
Ethics	Faith
Morals	Peace
Love	Fulfillment
Meaning and purpose	Connectedness

some individuals spirituality is related to religious beliefs, but that others develop spiritual health without belonging to organized religious groups. Spiritual health results in "a sense of inner peace and harmony" (p. 3).

At first this list of definitions and descriptions may seem to lack agreement. However, a closer look reveals common themes. Several include statements about values, ethics, or morals, or they list virtues such as love, forgiveness, faith, peace, and fulfillment. Several include statements about discovering life's meaning and purpose. The theme of connectedness is also apparent in these definitions and descriptions of spiritual health. This connectedness refers to our relationships with ourselves, others, the environment, and/or a higher power. However, a closer look reveals common themes (see **Box 6.1**).

Models of Spiritual Health

Models of spiritual health have been developed by a variety of writers. Three will be examined here. The first is a developmental model (Peck, 1987). Peck suggests that just as our bodies mature and develop, so does spiritual health. The other two models are component models. Banks (1980) and Seaward (1991, 1999) suggest there are identifiable characteristics of spiritually healthy individuals.

Stages of Spiritual Growth Model

The first model is a developmental model proposed by psychiatrist M. Scott Peck (1987). He describes four stages of spiritual growth: (1) chaotic, antisocial; (2) formal, institutional; (3) skeptic, individual; and finally (4) mystic, communal (see **Figure 6.2**). He believes the pattern is predictable but not inviolate. He also emphasizes that many people do not reach the final stage, and people sometimes revert to earlier stages.

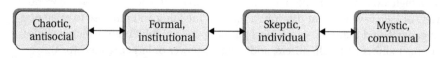

Figure 6.2 Peck's Model of Spiritual Health

CHAOTIC, ANTISOCIAL

Peck describes stage 1 of spiritual development as "undeveloped spirituality." People in the *chaotic, antisocial* stage are unable to love others; their relationships are "manipulative and self-serving." This is a chaotic time because the person lacks principles. Without principles to guide their lives, people in stage 1 act based on their immediate wants and desires. This leads to inconsistency and a lack of integrity. You never know what to expect from them. They may expect others to play fair, but have no qualms about deceiving others in order to fulfill their own desires. The only thing on the minds of people in stage 1 is their own needs. They are unaware of the needs of others.

FORMAL, INSTITUTIONAL

Sometimes people realize the chaos of their lives and decide they need to change. The transition into stage 2 is often a dramatic and sudden conversion experience. They realize they cannot continue to live as they have: "Anything is better than this." Addicts refer to this as "hitting bottom." At this point the person moves into stage 2, the *formal, institutional* stage of spiritual development. The person finds an *institution* (or a charismatic leader) to build a life around. The organization provides structure and clear guidelines for living. It may be prison, the military, a career, or religion. This stage is called *formal* because people cling to the rules, the expectations, and the forms of the institution or leader. People in the formal, institutional stage are uncomfortable with change because it seems chaotic. Therefore, they become very legalistic. There is "the right way" and any other way is "wrong." They have difficulty accepting that other perspectives may have some truth in them. The world is "black or white," "right or wrong," "my way or the highway."

SKEPTIC, INDIVIDUAL

Inevitably, institutions and leaders make mistakes or display a lack integrity. For some individuals, this leads to questions: "Can I really put my faith in this organization?" "If he says one thing but does another, how can I trust him?" These questions may lead a person into stage 3—the *skeptic, individual* stage. These individuals have enough self-confidence that they are no longer dependent on the institution that gave life meaning in stage 2. They begin to trust their own perceptions and beliefs. They make up their own minds on issues and feel capable of making decisions for themselves. People in stage 3 are individuals rather than followers in a group; however, this is not to say they are antisocial. They are often devoted to social causes such as feeding the hungry, saving the environment, or providing medical care to underserved individuals. They are active truth seekers.

MYSTIC, COMMUNAL

As stage 3 individuals begin to see bits and pieces of truth, they see the "big picture" in life and realize the world is amazingly beautiful. This marks the transition into stage 4, the *mystic, communal* stage. They often realize that the essential purpose and goals of the institution in stage 2 were true, even if the rules and rituals were not really essential. They begin to see the interconnectedness of all things. There is some unifying aspect to the world—somehow men, women, creatures, and inanimate objects are connected. A sense of community develops. There is mystery about this connection that motivates stage 4 individuals to seek greater understanding even though they know the mystery will grow as they learn more. The sense of mystery is attractive to them. They love questions, in contrast to demanding answers as they did in stage 2. Stage 4 individuals envision the entire world as a community.

This model proposes that the highest level of spiritual development is rare. It is characterized by appreciation of the mystery of life. Rather than being frightened by mystery, individuals in this stage embrace it. In addition, they feel connected to the world around them.

Banks's Model of Spiritual Health

The second model of spiritual health is based on a study conducted by Rebecca Banks (1980). Banks surveyed a sample of health educators several times to reach a consensus on four components of spiritual health. Based on this study she developed the following model. The four aspects she found were: (1) a unifying force within individuals, (2) meaning and purpose in life, (3) a bond between individuals, and (4) individual perceptions and faith.

UNIFYING FORCE

Spiritual health is the dimension that integrates the other dimensions. "Health" takes into account the whole person, and the spiritual dimension is the "central core" that provides a foundation for physical, social, emotional, and intellectual health. Thus, Banks's model of health places spiritual health at the center as the most important dimension.

MEANING AND PURPOSE IN LIFE

Identification of purpose in life is very personal. Victor Frankl (1963), a psychiatrist and concentration camp survivor, wrote that we must discover our own unique purpose. Once identified, however, this provides internal motivation for life's accomplishments. Purpose provides direction and allows you to live a fulfilling life.

BONDING BETWEEN INDIVIDUALS

Spiritual health transcends the individual. Spirituality provides the bond between individuals, particularly those who have identified similar purposes for their lives. It also transcends the physical universe and includes components such as belief in God or a higher power. This bonding also includes a sense of selflessness, empathy with others, and a set of principles to live by. Individuals are able to share warmth, love, and compassion.

INDIVIDUAL PERCEPTIONS AND FAITH

The spiritual dimension is the most difficult to quantify. Because faith is so individual, spirituality is quite subjective. Your beliefs about what causes the universe to function as it does and the recognition of powers beyond the "natural and rational" provide a foundation for faith. Religious faith is an aspect of this component as well.

Banks's model is based on the opinions of leading health educators. The model includes social aspects, faith in something bigger than self, and recognition of meaning in life. It also functions as a unifying force, providing a foundation for the other dimensions of health.

Seaward's Components of Spiritual Health

The third model was developed by Brian Luke Seaward (1991, 1999) from the University of Colorado at Boulder. He recognizes spiritual health as a process, and proposes three components that must be developed. Seaward (1999) defines spirituality as "the maturation process of our higher consciousness as developed through the integration of three facets: an insightful, nurturing relationship with oneself and others, the development of a strong personal value system, and a meaningful purpose in one's life" (p. 150). Each facet is "mutually inclusive of the other two." They overlap and interact; for example, values influence one's purpose in life.

INTERNAL AND EXTERNAL RELATIONSHIPS

The first component is relationships. Seaward (1999) believes that two types of relationships contribute to spiritual health. The first type is internal, your relationship with yourself. He believes that you must nurture yourself in order to develop spiritually. This requires time alone. Solitude allows the opportunity for self-discovery and separating who you are from what you do and who your friends are. Seaward compares developing your internal relationship to Jung's concept of individuation, the process of developing a personal identity. Jung, an influential psychiatrist, recommended self-reflection and soul-searching in order to develop intuition, creativity, willpower, faith, patience, optimism, and humbleness (Seaward, 1999). This process results in the ability to accept and love yourself.

The second type of relationship is external. This includes health-enhancing relationships with family, friends, and acquaintances, as well as the environment. Seaward (1999) suggests that we can develop external relationships through respect for and acceptance of others, as well as feelings of connectedness to nature. Healthy external relationships are characterized by tolerance, acceptance, and respect for the opinions, beliefs, and values of others even when they contradict your own. He reminds us of the Golden Rule that is present in some form in all major religions, "Do unto others as you would have them do unto you."

He suggests that both types of relationships require continual attention. Relationships are dynamic and need constant care and feeding.

PERSONAL VALUE SYSTEM

The second component of Seaward's model is your personal value system. Values are "personal beliefs based on the concepts of good, justice, and beauty that give meaning and depth to your thoughts, attitudes, and behaviors" (Seaward, 1999, p. 151). Values are often learned during childhood from parents, teachers, and other significant adults. As children grow, value conflicts are inevitable. As we experience more in life our childhood values may be challenged. This results in a process of maturation as values are modified and develop more fully. Resolving value conflicts requires work, but the results are very rewarding.

MEANINGFUL PURPOSE IN LIFE

Meaningful purpose in life is the third component of Seaward's (1999) model. He cites Frankl's belief that the search for meaning is a primary force and instinctual for humans (Frankl, 1963). Finding new goals throughout life is a crucial aspect of developing a "life mission." When a major portion of life ends (e.g., school or parenting), a period of questioning and suffering may occur as we search for a new mission.

Seaward's (1999) model suggests that the three components yield specific personality traits or resources that, when expressed, result in spiritual health. These traits include creativity, will, intuition, faith, patience, courage, love, humility, and optimism. Even when these traits are dormant they reflect spiritual potential.

Obstacles to spiritual development exist. These roadblocks include laziness, greed, despair, addictions, and low self-esteem. They slow the maturation process and prevent you from reaching your potential. Thankfully, there are activities that can enhance spiritual development. Seaward (1999) calls these activities interventions. You can use these consciously to improve your spiritual health. Meditation, relaxation techniques, and the arts are recommended interventions.

Both Peck's (1987) developmental and Seaward's (1999) component models emphasize relationships and the search for meaning. These characteristics are evidence of spiritual health.

Characteristics of the Spiritually Healthy Person

How can we recognize high levels of spiritual health? What can we do to develop spiritually? Several authors have made suggestions to help us answer these questions.

Chapman (1987) writes that "optimal spiritual health . . . would include our ability to discover and articulate our own basic purpose in life, learn how to experience love, joy, peace, and fulfillment, and how to help ourselves and others achieve their full potential" (p. 32).

Scandurra (1999) believes that we need to recognize the connection between everyday activities and spiritual health. She suggests journaling, mindfulness practice, meditation, and yoga as such activities.

Turner, Sizer, Whitney, and Wilks (1992) developed a scale to assess spiritual health. Activities that indicate higher levels of spirituality include spending time with people who are different from you, attending religious services, helping the needy, enjoying nature, reading inspirational writings, meditating, praying, and enjoying the arts. To further develop the spiritual dimension they recommend keeping a journal, praying and meditating regularly, cultivating humility and a sense of oneness with others, and being open to messages about how to live your life.

Strategies for enhancing spiritual health are also proposed by Hales (2005) in her health textbook. She recommends attending religious services or joining a prayer group. For those who are not religious she suggests keeping an open mind about religion and spirituality, as well as reading the writings of people of faith (e.g., Martin Luther King, Jr. or Mohandas Gandhi). Secular activities include meditation and stress management techniques, spending time with wise people, and enjoying nature.

Physician N. Lee Smith (Donatelle, 2005) suggests that you can recognize spiritual health in the following ways: (1) you are at peace with yourself and "in good standing with the environment," (2) you have a sense of empowerment and control that includes feeling valued, (3) you feel connected to your innermost self and to others, (4) you have a sense of purpose in your life, (5) you enjoy growing and have a sense of your potential, and (6) you have a sense of hope for the future. Thomas and Kotecki (2007, p. 7) also suggest components of spiritual health: "selflessness, compassion, a passion for living, faith, a sense of right and wrong, ethics, and morals."

Steven Hawks (1994) from Utah State University suggests that spiritually healthy people have a clear worldview and exhibit faith, hope, and commitment based on that worldview. He also believes the spiritually well feel connected with themselves, others, and some higher power or "larger reality."

A New Model of Spiritual Health

Examination of the definitions and models presented above reveals some common themes. All three models include relationships or connectedness. Peck's (1987) highest level of spiritual development includes community. Banks (1980) refers to a willingness to do more for others than for yourself. Seaward (1991, 1999) includes both internal and external relationships in his three-component model.

References to ethics, values, and morals are also common. Some authors list virtues such as love, faith, forgiveness, and hope. Most people believe that a virtuous life builds character.

The third common theme is fulfillment, meaning, and purpose in life. Most definitions refer to this characteristic. Breuss and Richardson (1994) suggest that lack of purpose is a feature of poor spiritual health. The models of both Banks (1980) and Seaward (1991, 1999) incorporate meaning and purpose.

Taken together the following three themes comprise our model of spiritual health: (1) character and virtue, (2) meaning and purpose, and (3) connectedness (see **Figure 6.3**).

Character and Virtue

Living in harmony with principles (or virtues) develops character. The virtues provide guidelines for living effectively with yourself and with others. In his book *Authentic Happiness*, psychologist Martin Seligman (2002) writes that issues

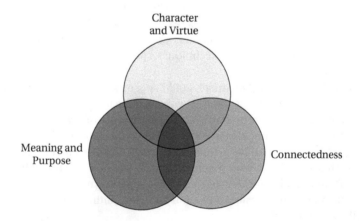

Figure 6.3 A Model of Spiritual Health

of character were largely ignored (at least in psychology) during the twentieth century. During that time the belief was that behavior could be explained by one's environment rather than by something within the individual. "Bad" behavior resulted from a "bad" environment, and vice versa. More recently people have begun to reconsider this hypothesis.

Covey (1989) also believes that the importance of character has been diminished. His review of the "success literature" over the past 150 years reveals a trend toward a "personality ethic"; that is, people depend on techniques and behaviors (sometimes even tricks) when dealing with life and other people. However, prior to the twentieth century, it was assumed that behavior was an outgrowth of character. This "character ethic" assumes that there is something within each person that plays a role in behavior.

Seligman (2002) and his colleagues believe that ignoring character has come at a cost. They set out to examine character. They studied writings from the major religious and philosophical traditions and identified 200 "virtue catalogues" written over a period of 3,000 years in cultures around the world. They identified six ubiquitous virtues: (1) wisdom and knowledge, (2) courage, (3) love and humanity, (4) justice, (5) temperance, and (6) spirituality and transcendence. These six virtues are the "core characteristics endorsed by almost all religious and philosophical traditions, and taken together they capture the notion of good character" (Seligman, 2002, p. 133).

Let's take a moment to develop a better understanding of two crucial terms we have been using: character and virtue. Both of these terms are abstract, making it difficult to agree on precise definitions; however, we can develop a working understanding of each concept. Character is about "*knowing* the good, *loving* the good, and *doing* the good" (Ryan & Bohlin, 1999, p. 5). Thomas Lickona (2004), a developmental psychologist and leader of character education programs in schools, writes, "We need character to lead purposeful, productive, and fulfilling lives. . . . We need character to build a civil, decent, and just society" (p. xxii). Character is the composite of our good habits, called virtues, and our bad habits, known as vices. Virtues dominate in people of good character.

Virtues are "dispositions to behave in a morally good way" (Lickona, 2004, p. 7). As mentioned earlier, they are qualities that are affirmed by societies and religions around the world. For individuals of high character, virtues promote happiness and satisfaction with life. According to Lickona, virtues meet the ethical tests of reversibility and universalizability. Reversibility asks, "If you reverse the situation, is this the way you would like to be treated?" A virtue is universal if you would want all persons to act this way in a similar situation. Let's examine the ubiquitous virtues identified by Seligman (2002).

Wisdom requires knowledge. The ancient Greeks considered wisdom to be the "master virtue" because it directs all the other virtues (Lickona, 2004). Wise people possess the knowledge and the inclination to make decisions that are good both for themselves and for others. The wise person displays empathy and realizes the consequences of decisions in advance. Wisdom enables us to set priorities. Seligman (2002) suggests that there are several paths to wisdom. Curiosity opens new ideas and worlds to us. The curious are open-minded, able to set aside preconceived notions when evidence contradicts them. People naturally love learning, and this opens another path. Have you ever been around a 2- or 3-year-old who asks questions about everything? "Why is the sky blue?" "Why is thunder so loud?" Curiosity and love of learning are closely related. Wise people make sound judgments based on accurate information. They think of consequences and alternatives.

Courage is sometimes referred to as fortitude. Courage is the virtue that enables us to do right even when it is difficult. A woman at an Alcoholics Anonymous meeting once described recovery as a series of choices. You have the easy, alcoholic choice or the difficult, healthy choice (Knapp, 1996). If someone has the answers to an exam, it takes courage for you to say, "No thanks. I'll see what I can do on my own." It would be easy to look at the answers, especially in this day when grades are emphasized at every level of education. Courage requires integrity and commitment to higher ideals. It requires perspective, a long-term view.

Justice is often apparent in civic activities (Seligman, 2002). Strengths that develop justice include citizenship, duty, fairness, equity, and leadership. We usually think of citizenship in the context of our home country, but we are also citizens of smaller groups. When you work in a small group for a class, you are a citizen of that group. In the interest of justice (as well as wisdom and knowledge), you must do your duty. If some work is due on Tuesday, you need to complete it so the group can move forward. You must function as a team member thinking of the good of the group rather than yourself. If you have leadership skills and qualities, you must contribute them to the group by organizing and supervising the other team members.

Love is a social virtue. It exists in the context of human relationships. Love is different from justice. Justice requires fairness; love offers more. It is a willingness to sacrifice your own wants and desires for someone else. Love appears in both the ordinary and the extraordinary. It is in the ordinary when you are willing to order a pizza without your favorite topping because your date doesn't like it. Love is apparent in the extraordinary when a father gives his own life to save his child. "Love your neighbor as yourself" is a concept that exists in virtually every civilization. Lickona (2004) suggests several supporting virtues related to love: empathy, compassion, kindness, generosity, service, loyalty, and forgiveness. The underlying motivation for love is recognition of the inherent worth of another human being.

Temperance is often a misunderstood virtue. The term is seldom used in conversation. If it is used, it is probably in the context of controlling one's alcohol consumption. However, the concept is much broader. Some name this virtue *self-control*. Temperance requires the discipline to govern yourself, to control your temper, to regulate your appetites, and to pursue pleasure in moderation. The temperate person is able to take a long-term view, to delay gratification for more important goals in the future.

The sixth ubiquitous virtue identified by Seligman (2002) is *transcendence*. Transcendence refers to "emotional strengths that reach outside and beyond you to connect you to something larger and more permanent" (Seligman, p. 154). Transcendence is apparent when you are overwhelmed by a sunset or a rainbow. Transcendence occurs when you witness or participate in an outstanding athletic event or a beautiful concert. When you feel gratitude for the good things in your life, such as family, friends, or wisdom, you are experiencing transcendence. Forgiveness is also transcending, as is hope in the future and a zest for life. Recognition that God loves you is another example of transcendence.

Virtuous living contributes to the "good life." Seligman (2002) believes there are multiple paths to achieve each virtue. He names these paths, or subvirtues, character strengths and suggests that you take the time to identify your personal strengths. Once you know your strengths, you can begin to incorporate them into your life. Thomas Aquinas described two aspects of virtue (Dunnam & Reisman, 1998): habit and power. We are not born virtuous; it takes training. We develop the virtues through practice. If we want to be just, we must act justly. We must make a habit of living virtuously. Living a virtuous life gives us power to make a difference, to change the world (or at least our part of it) for the better.

Meaning and Purpose

The second component of spiritual health is to identify meaning and purpose in your life. Covey, Merrill, and Merrill (1994) make a distinction between living by the clock and living by the compass. People who live by the clock focus on efficiency, on getting a lot done. Those who live by the compass have identified what is most important in their lives and live by priorities. The compass provides direction, meaning, and purpose. We often get caught up in the "activity trap" where we mistake busy-ness for productivity and value. Identifying our purpose in life gives direction and helps us set priorities. Our actions then follow and will be congruent with our purpose.

Naylor, Willimon, and Naylor (1994) taught an undergraduate seminar on finding meaning in life at Duke University. Their book is a compilation of things learned during that seminar. They believe that meaning is "perhaps the central problem of modern people" (p. 7). They cite data regarding alcohol abuse, rape, and the desire for wealth as evidence of meaninglessness among America's college students. Students who want to grow up to be "moneymaking machines" are described as the "living dead." The authors suggest that there are more important aspects to living a good, meaningful life. They suggest that we must ask important questions in order to discover meaning and purpose. The questions are classic questions of philosophy: Why am I here? Where am I going? Who am I? What is the purpose of life? Is there a God?

People whose lives are meaningless often suffer despair and depression. In contrast, people who have discovered meaning experience growth and balance as a result of their quest. Naylor and colleagues (1994) suggest that we need to focus on *being* rather than *having* or *accumulating*, and that we need to develop a personal philosophy and strategy. Covey (1994) calls this individual philosophy a personal mission statement. A formal mission statement is important because it brings clarity, focus, and discipline to our lives.

Finding meaning and purpose is a search, a process that continues throughout life. Naylor, Willimon, and Naylor (1994) suggest that there are various pathways to meaning; however, they suggest that virtually all of them include our "need for human love and empathy and our intense longing for community" (p. 26). We need to consider the legacy we want to leave on earth when we are gone.

Connectedness

Connectedness refers to your relationships. When you are spiritually healthy you are in touch with yourself, those around you, the environment, and the eternal. Seaward (2001) refers to personal connectedness as an internal relationship. It is closely related to the virtues because it includes self-discipline and self-governance. Knowing yourself requires introspection and reflection. A central theme of your internal relationship is recognition that you are part of something bigger. This leads to your external relationships, those with other individuals and your environment. You recognize that you play a role in life that is bigger and grander than caring for yourself. This includes citizenship, as well as friendship. It is societal and interpersonal.

Stephen Covey (1989) proposed a pattern for living in his book *The 7 Habits of Highly Effective People*. The first three habits lead to "private victories." The goal is to become effective individuals. Private victories develop character. People of character are able to develop productive relationships with others. Covey emphasizes that you do not have to have a perfect internal relationship before you can work on external relationships, which he labels "public victories." He proposes three habits to enhance relationships with those around you. First, you must think win/win. What is best for all involved? Next, you must understand the needs and desires of others. This is empathy. Empathy is more than just hearing; it is understanding the content, the context, and the feelings of others. Finally, you seek unique solutions that meet the needs of all the stakeholders. You watch out for yourself and others equally. You feel connected to others in your life.

Peck's (1987) model of spiritual development also emphasizes connectedness. At the highest level, spirituality is communal. Peck does not use the term *communal* lightly; community is not just a group of people who inhabit the same place or share some common interest. Community has three characteristics that emphasize connectedness. First, community is inclusive. People seeking community are motivated to include others, even those who act, think, or feel differently. Second, community requires commitment. Inclusion is possible only when people are committed to the group. There must be a "willingness to coexist." You have to hang in there even if you feel excluded or that the community isn't meeting your needs. Consensus is the third prerequisite for community. People learn to appreciate, even celebrate, differences. Recognizing differences means that decisions must be made for the good of all. This occurs when all members recognize the value and importance of everyone in the group. Connectedness creates a climate in which discussion and debate contribute to an understanding of the highest good for the group and its individuals. When these three conditions of connectedness are present, community, "a group that has learned to transcend its individual differences," exists (Peck, 1987, p. 62). Naylor, Willimon, and Naylor (1994) believe that "through community we can show empathy for another's search for meaning by suspending our own frame of reference so that we may confront the spiritual, intellectual, and emotional world of the other" (p. 128).

High levels of spiritual health exist among people of character who feel connected to the people around them and have identified meaning and purpose in their lives. This forms the core of their being.

Conclusion

Spiritually healthy people recognize a purpose in life. Something greater than themselves provides meaning. These people also feel a sense of belonging, a connectedness, to the world around them. Their concern for that world leads them to act virtuously. They care.

Discussion Questions

1. Name someone or something to which you feel connected. Explain the connection.
2. Examine the virtues described earlier. Describe one recent virtuous act you have committed.
3. Identify an individual whom you admire. What virtues does he or she exhibit?
4. Think about what provides meaning for your life. Describe the significance of that aspect of your life.

References

Alters, S., & Schiff, W. (2009). *Essential concepts for healthy living* (5th ed.). Sudbury, MA: Jones and Bartlett.

Banks, R. (1980). Health and the spiritual dimension: Relationships and implications for professional preparation programs. *Journal of School Health, 50*(4), 195–202.

Barnhart, R. K. (ed.). (1988). *The Barnhart dictionary of etymology.* New York: H.W. Wilson.

Bensley, R. J. (1991). Defining spiritual health: A review of the literature. *Journal of Health Education, 22*(5), 287–297.

Bloomfield, H., & Kory, R. (1978). *The holistic way to health and happiness.* New York: Simon & Schuster.

Breuss, C. E., & Richardson, G. E. (1994). *Healthy decisions.* Madison, WI: Brown & Benchmark.

Byer, C. O., & Shainberg, L. W. (1995). *Living well: Health in your hands* (2nd ed.). New York: Harper Collins College.

Chantrell, C. (ed.). (2002). *The Oxford dictionary of word histories.* Oxford: Oxford University Press.

Chapman, L. (1987). Developing a useful perspective on spiritual health: Well-being, spiritual potential and the search for meaning. *American Journal of Health Promotion, 1*(3), 31–39.

Covey, S. R. (1989). *The 7 habits of highly effective people.* New York: Simon & Schuster.

Covey, S. R., Merrill, A. R., & Merrill, R .R. (1994). *First things first.* New York: Simon & Schuster.

Donatelle, R. (2005). *Health: The basics* (6th ed.). San Francisco: Pearson Benjamin Cummings.

Dunnam, M., & Reisman, K. D. (1998). *The workbook on virtues and the fruit of the spirit.* Nashville, TN: Upper Room.

Floyd, P. A., Mimms, S. E., & Yelding, C. (2008). *Personal health: Perspectives and lifestyles* (4th ed.). Belmont, CA: Thomson Wadsworth.

Frankl, V. E. (1963). *Man's search for meaning.* New York: Washington Square Press.

Hales, D. (2005). *An invitation to health* (11th ed.). Belmont, CA: Thomson Wadsworth.

Hales, D. (2009). *An invitation to health* (12th ed.). Belmont, CA: Wadsworth Cengage Learning.

Hawks, S. (1994). Spiritual health: Definition and theory. *Wellness Perspectives, 10*(4), 3–13.

Insel, P. M., & Roth, W. T. (2004). *Core concepts in health* (9th ed.). Boston: McGraw-Hill.

Knapp, C. (1996). *Drinking: A love story.* New York: Dial Press.

Lickona, T. (2004). *Character matters: How to help our children develop good judgment, integrity, and other essential virtues.* New York: Touchstone.

Naylor, T. H., Willimon, W. H., & Naylor, M. R. (1994). *The search for meaning.* Nashville, TN: Abingdon Press.

Peck, M. S. (1987). *The different drum: Community making and peace.* New York: Simon & Schuster.

Russell, R. (1987). If I were a rich man . . . health education. *Eta Sigma Gamman, 19*(2), 39–41.

Ryan, K., & Bohlin, K. E. (1999). *Building character in school: Practical ways to bring moral instruction to life.* San Francisco: Jossey-Bass.

Scandurra, D. J. (1999). Everyday spirituality: A core unit in health education and lifetime wellness. *Journal of Health Education, 30*(2), 104–109.

Seaward, B. L. (1991). Spiritual wellbeing: A health education model. *Journal of Health Education, 22*(3), 166–169.

Seaward, B. L. (1999). *Managing stress: Principles and strategies for health and wellbeing.* Sudbury, MA: Jones and Bartlett.

Seaward, B. L. (2001). *Health of the human spirit: Spiritual dimensions for personal health.* Boston: Allyn and Bacon.

Seligman, M. E. P. (2002). *Authentic happiness.* New York: Free Press.

Thomas, D. Q., & Kotecki, J. E. (2007). *Physical activity and health: An interactive approach* (2nd ed.). Sudbury, MA: Jones and Bartlett.

Turner, L. W., Sizer, F. S., Whitney, E. N., & Wilks, B. B. (1992). *Life choices: Health concepts and strategies* (2nd ed.). St. Paul, MN: West.

Young, E. (1984). Spiritual health—an essential element in optimum health. *Journal of American College Health, 32*, 273–276.

CHAPTER 7 ▶

Health: Wrapping It Up

We are wholes. Body, mind, and soul.

—George Sheehan, 1992

Health lies not in the parts but in the whole.

—Carl E. and LaVonne Braaten, 1976

Health is a multidimensional concept that continues to evolve. The five dimensions of health are overlapping and interacting. Identifying distinct dimensions allows organized study of health, but in reality, health is a unified whole. The healthy individual functions at peak levels. Health, however, is not static. It is fluid. Sometimes we experience high-level wellness. At other times one or more dimensions are impaired. When one dimension is affected, the others are impacted as well. If you break a leg, your ability to move, to think, to serve, and to love may be altered.

The value of analyzing each dimension of health is to understand the components of health and recognize their overlapping, interacting nature. **Figure 7.1** illustrates this relationship. We see the whole shape but also the overlapping dimensions. The space in the center represents the highest level of health, a condition in which all five dimensions are in harmony.

This chapter will use two scenarios to illustrate the overlapping, interacting nature of the dimensions of health. The first scenario examines college life in general and how it can affect health. The second examines a student's response to the end of a relationship—a break-up.

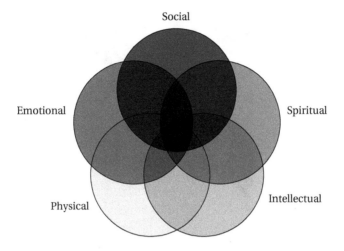

Figure 7.1 The Dimensions of Health

College Life

Life at college can be like riding a roller coaster. The highs and lows affect all aspects of life and health. Caroline enrolled at her first-choice college, intending to pursue a degree in business and finance. Her career goal was to join a successful company, earn quick promotions, and make a lot of money. Although she probably would not have expressed it this way, her motive for attending college was to learn what she needed to get rich. She knew she needed to master the required material and earn a degree in order to enter her chosen field.

Caroline's mother developed breast cancer during Caroline's first year of college. This time of uncertainty affected Caroline's emotional health as she experienced fear and anxiety. She used her fears to learn about cancer and the available treatments. When the cancer went into remission, Caroline experienced joy and relief. After this experience she felt connected to people suffering from cancer. She also began to realize that there are many ways to use a business degree. She developed a desire to help cure cancer and realized that she could use her education to further this goal through fundraising efforts. This demonstrates a direct correlation with spiritual health—a sense of purpose. Caroline's spiritual and intellectual health complemented each other.

As Caroline's intellectual health developed, her emotional health was also affected. She experienced pride in her academic accomplishments. However, Caroline became so involved in her studies and her internship that she became isolated. She did not date or develop new friendships. Eventually she realized that she was lonely and began to spend more time with her roommates and other

Participation in events such as Race for the Cure illustrates the overlapping, interacting nature of the dimensions of health.

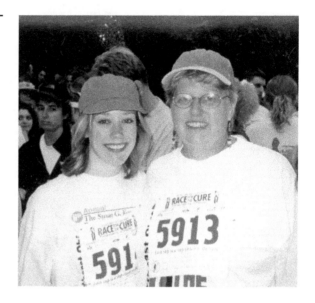

friends. She found the discussions stimulating and discovered that she could share her deepest thoughts with her roommate. Caroline also found that her friends supported her goals, and some even became involved in cancer awareness and fundraising activities with her.

Caroline's university required a personal health class as part of the general education program. Caroline realized that lifestyle choices affect health, including her own risk of cancer. Learning about the body and applying that knowledge to her own life improved her health. She began to exercise regularly and choose her foods more carefully. The interaction of physical and intellectual health helped Caroline reduce risks of disease and increase energy levels. She learned how to take care of her body in order to perform at optimal levels.

College life required Caroline to interact with professors and fellow students. Often professors assigned group work in order to develop interpersonal skills. This ability to work with others is often necessary in the workplace. Caroline was required on several occasions to develop business or marketing plans in small group activities. As she learned about the topic she also developed listening and negotiating skills, which improved her social health. She learned to recognize and deal constructively with the frustration that occurs when trying to meet deadlines and work with both less motivated and highly opinionated classmates.

An individual's health changes over time. External events such as illness can affect health positively or negatively. The cancer caused emotional turmoil, but also stimulated intellectual activity. Caroline's experience with her mother's illness also shaped her purpose in life, and this improved her spiritual health. She became more concerned with others and less concerned with her financial security. As this example demonstrates, health is a dynamic condition.

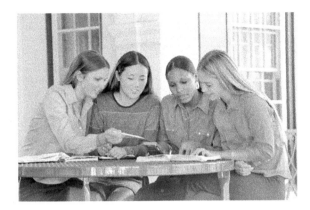

Working in small groups can improve social, emotional, and intellectual health.

The Break-up

Sometimes short-term situations affect health, too. Kelly and Ted had been dating each other exclusively for 2 years. About this time, Ted realized he wasn't ready for such a serious relationship. He decided he should break up with Kelly. Kelly was shocked by his announcement. She felt abandoned and misled. She couldn't stop wondering what went wrong. She couldn't sleep, had no appetite, and lost interest in her schoolwork. She just wanted to be alone with her thoughts. Luckily her friends recognized her distress and provided support for her. As Kelly recovered from this change in her life, she began to consider what she wanted from her life. She began to ask the "big questions." She realized that her life had value and purpose even without Ted.

This scenario illustrates multiple overlaps among the dimensions of health. Initially Kelly's social health deteriorated as an important relationship ended suddenly. This change had a negative effect on her physical health as she slept poorly and ate little. Her emotional health suffered as she felt anger toward Ted and despair as she questioned her own worth. Kelly's apathy toward school also affected her intellectual health. She lacked motivation to learn the necessary material for her classes.

On the positive side, Kelly had strong friendships. Her friends rallied around her and helped her move ahead with her life. Their support was crucial. As Kelly recovered she found this change in her circumstances gave her a chance to reevaluate her life. She discovered that her identity was bigger than just being "Ted's girlfriend." She began to volunteer at a local community center and found that this type of service was very rewarding. Looking outside herself and caring for others represented an improvement in her spiritual health. Humans are remarkably resilient. Kelly discovered this as she lived through a difficult experience. From this example, we can see how one situation can affect different dimensions of health.

Conclusion

Health is a lifelong process. This process requires the individual to care for the body, to develop and maintain uplifting relationships, to recognize and

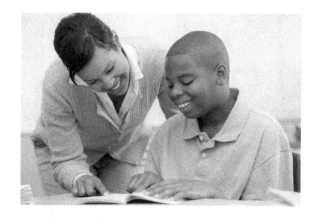

Helping others improves spiritual health.

constructively express a full range of emotions, to learn and apply knowledge to help oneself and one's community, and to recognize and act on one's meaning and purpose in life. The healthy person feels connected to the surrounding world. This connectedness includes the environment, strangers and friends, and God.

Feeling connected to those around you enhances health.

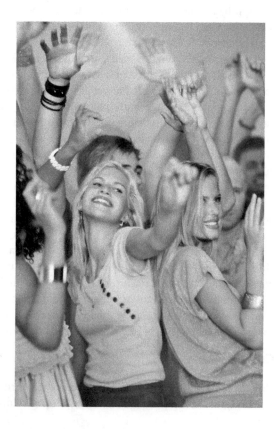

The healthy individual functions at optimal levels. Health is a holistic concept. It is concerned with the whole person. Five components or dimensions comprise the whole. These five dimensions are overlapping and interacting. When one dimension is altered, the others change as well. Therefore, it is important to exercise the "dimensions of our nature regularly and consistently in wise and balanced ways" (Covey, 1989, p. 289). So live life fully and enjoy good health. *Carpe diem!*

Discussion Questions

1. Describe an incident in your life that demonstrates the overlapping, interacting nature of the dimensions of health.
2. Describe how exercise can affect more than one dimension of health.
3. Describe how a good meal can affect more than one dimension of health.
4. If you had to choose one dimension as the most important, which would it be? Why?

Reference

Covey, S. R. (1989). *The 7 habits of highly effective people: Powerful lessons in personal change.* New York: Fireside.

INDEX

Photo Credits

Chapter 1

Page 5 © Nicholas Piccillo/ShutterStock, Inc.; **page 6** © MarFot/ShutterStock, Inc.

Chapter 2

Page 9 (top left) © JHogan/ShutterStock, Inc.; **page 9 (top right)** © Jack Hollingsworth/Dreamstime.com; **page 9 (middle left)** © Anton Albert/Shutter-Stock, Inc.; **page 9 (bottom left)** © Photoeuphoria/Dreamstime.com; **page 9 (bottom right)** © Rmarmion/Dreamstime.com; **page 12 (top left)** © AbleStock; **page 12 (top right)** © Alfred Wekelo/ShutterStock, Inc.; **page 12 (bottom left)** © Losevsky Pavel/ShutterStock, Inc.; **page 12 (bottom right)** © Photodisc; **page 13 (left)** © Morgan Lane Photography/ShutterStock, Inc.; **page 13 (right)** © Photodisc; **page 17** © Photodisc; **page 20** © Photodisc; **page 21** © LiquidLibrary

Chapter 3

Page 25 (top) © NorthGeorgiaMedia/ShutterStock, Inc.; **page 25 (bottom)** © Photodisc; **page 28** © Feverpitch/ShutterStock, Inc.; **page 30** © Christina Richards/ShutterStock, Inc.; **page 33** © Geoffrey Kuchera/Dreamstime.com

Chapter 4

Page 37 (top left) © Lee Morris/ShutterStock, Inc.; **page 37 (top right)** © Galina Barskaya/ShutterStock, Inc.; **page 37 (middle left)** © Uschi Hering/Shutter-Stock, Inc.; **page 37 (middle right)** © Photos.com; **page 37 (bottom)** © Mark Fairey/Dreamstime.com; **page 39 (left)** © AbleStock; **page 39 (right)** © Sean Nel/ShutterStock, Inc.; **page 41** © June Steward/ShutterStock, Inc.

Chapter 5

Page 52 (bottom) © Can Balcioglu/Dreamstime.com; **page 54** © Lisa F. Young/ShutterStock, Inc.; **page 61** © Olga Lyubkina/Dreamstime.com

Chapter 6

Page 69 © Dreamstime Agency/Dreamstime.com; **page 71** © Sam DCruz/ShutterStock, Inc.

Chapter 7

Page 88 Courtesy of David Emanuel; **page 89** © LiquidLibrary; **page 90 (top)** © Monkey Business Images/ShutterStock, Inc.; **page 90 (bottom)** © Yuri Arcurs/Dreamstime.com

Unless otherwise indicated, all photographs and illustrations are under copyright of Jones and Bartlett Publishers, LLC.

CPSIA information can be obtained
at www.ICGtesting.com
Printed in the USA
BVHW052137180123
656542BV00015BA/716